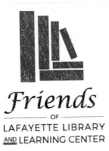

Hello
Sleep

Contents

Contents

FOR MY FATHER,
WHO INSPIRED ME TO PURSUE SCIENCE,

AND MY MOTHER,
WHO TAUGHT ME TO WRITE

Names and identifying characteristics of individuals discussed in the text
have been changed to protect the privacy of patients.

The information in this book is not intended to replace the advice of the reader's own
physician or other medical professional. You should consult a medical professional in matters
relating to health, especially if you have existing medical conditions, and before starting,
stopping, or changing the dose of any medication you are taking. Individual readers are
solely responsible for their own health-care decisions. The author and the publisher do not
accept responsibility for any adverse effects individuals may claim to experience, whether
directly or indirectly, from the information contained in this book.

First published in the United States by St. Martin's Essentials,
an imprint of St. Martin's Publishing Group

www.stmartins.com

Designed by Michelle McMillian

Library of Congress Cataloging-in-Publication Data

Names: Wu, Jade (Sleep psychologist), author.
Title: Hello sleep : the science and art of overcoming insomnia without
    medications / Jade Wu, Ph.D..
Description: First edition. | New York : St. Martin's Essentials, 2023. |
    Includes bibliographical references and index.
Identifiers: LCCN 2022045387 | ISBN 9781250828408 (hardcover) |
    ISBN 9781250828415 (ebook)
Subjects: LCSH: Sleep—Popular works. | Sleep disorders—Popular works.
Classification: LCC RA786 .W8 2023 | DDC 616.8/498—dc23/eng/20220920
LC record available at https://lccn.loc.gov/2022045387

Our books may be purchased in bulk for promotional, educational, or business use.
Please contact your local bookseller or the Macmillan Corporate and Premium
Sales Department at 1-800-221-7945, extension 5442, or by email at
MacmillanSpecialMarkets@macmillan.com.

First Edition: 2023

10   9   8   7   6   5   4   3   2

Hello
Sleep

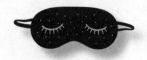

The Science and Art of Overcoming
Insomnia Without Medications

JADE WU, PhD

ST. MARTIN'S
ESSENTIALS
NEW YORK

Sleep Is a Friend,
Not an Engineering Problem

When I first met Kate, she had a wild look in her eyes. When I asked her what brought her to the Duke Behavioral Sleep Medicine Clinic, her voice cracked. She told me, "My sleep is broken. And I'm so, so tired."

Kate was a petite woman in her midforties with an easy smile and a mane of luxurious blonde hair. I could tell at first glance that she was all business. She had arrived before the clinic opened, clutching a laptop bag and thick folio of papers. She looked like a pint-sized Erin Brockovich ready to tackle her toughest case.

In a way, Kate *was* a detective. By day she worked as a software engineer, but by night she devoted her time to catching the thief who had stolen her sleep.

The folio she carried, it turned out, contained four months' worth of data she had amassed, including nightly sleep stats, daily food and drink intake, stress level fluctuations, and a record of her daily activities. It was an impressive compendium of evidence, complete with graphs and summary statistics. She was trying to find some pattern, some spark of understanding, that would crack the code of where her sleep had gone. My heart went out to her—she was working so hard!

But her investigation had hit a dead end.

Kate explained that some four years ago she had gone through a stressful time at work. She was answering emails at 11:00 P.M. to placate an unreasonable boss, and as part of an ultracompetitive team, was always made to feel like she could be fired at any time. Understandably, she started having trouble falling asleep because she would mentally plan work tasks for the next day or worry about some snide remark a coworker had made. At some point, almost imperceptibly, "insomnia" snuck into the vocabulary of her life.

But even after starting a new job where she felt valued, could flex her creativity, and enjoy her team's supportive culture, her ability to sleep somehow continued to get worse.

By the time I met her, it was taking Kate at least one to two hours to fall asleep on most nights. She no longer had work worries, but her mind always managed to churn anyway, even if it was just replaying a Christmas song for the seventeenth time. After tossing and turning and desperately trying to shut down her mind, she'd eventually fall into a fitful sleep. But she would only stay asleep for three hours before waking up again, and again, and again . . . every hour, on the hour. She would get up in the morning feeling like she'd been run over by a truck.

Kate is not alone. She might have been exceptional in her devotion to data-gathering, but the agony of her nighttime hours is something legions of the sleepless understand. While insomnia is one of the loneliest human experiences, it's also nearly universal. Almost everyone has a bout of sleeplessness at some point in life, and a surprisingly large number end up struggling with it for years or even decades.

You may be one of the chronically sleepless. Even if you feel alone in

the impenetrable night, know that 24.5 million other American adults*
are also wondering if they're losing their mind, if the sleep center of their
brain is broken. Perhaps, like them, you manage to get through the day,
but it feels as if you're dragging your feet through mud and your brain
through molasses. Perhaps, like Kate, you snap at your kids when you
don't mean to because insomnia has shortened your fuse and frayed your
edges. Then you spend the rest of the day feeling both tired *and* guilty.

Perhaps, like so many others, you feel that sleep has betrayed you.

At one point during our first conversation, Kate threw up her hands
and exclaimed, "And the craziest thing is—I can't even nap! Sometimes
I'm so exhausted and I just want to curl up and catch ten minutes. Not
asking for too much, right? But I lie there wide awake until I'm too frustrated to keep trying."

"It sounds like you're tired but wired during the day?" I asked.

"Exactly. And this is in the evenings too. Sometimes I'm actually nodding off on the couch while watching TV, and I think that if I just go *veeeery*
quietly to bed, I'll trick my brain into keeping on sleeping. But nope. As
soon as I lie down in bed, it's like a switch flips on. And from there it's just
busy, busy, busy in my head. Why is my brain *doing* this to me?"

Why, indeed? What had Kate (and what have you) done to deserve
this? You go to bed at a decent hour. You worship caffeine in the mornings but avoid it like the plague after noon. You manage stress as well
as one can (other than the whole not-sleeping thing). You follow all the
sleep hygiene rules better than you've followed any diet. You bought
an expensive mattress and tried three different brands of melatonin, or
perhaps prescription drugs like Ambien or Lunesta. You meditate like
your life depends on it.

---

* J. G. Ellis, M. L. Perlis, L. F. Neale, C. A. Espie, and C. H. Bastien, "The Natural History of Insomnia:
Focus on Prevalence and Incidence of Acute Insomnia," *Journal of Psychiatric Research* 46, no. 10 (2012):
1278–85.

Or maybe you haven't been perfect in any of these domains, but then again, why should you be? Sleep shouldn't be this hard, right?

You've somehow lost control of sleep. And like Kate, all you want to do is figure out *why,* and *how* this happened, and most important, how you can get it back in line. Should you stop looking at electronic screens by 8:00 P.M.? (Spoiler: nope, you don't need to do that.) Should you buy special white noise machines, or Himalayan salt lamps, or lavender mist, or a wearable sleep tracker with the latest features? (Nope. That may backfire.) Should you make sure to be in bed at the same time every night? (Definitely nope. That will surely backfire.) Should you try melatonin again? (You could, but it won't help.)

So, what's the answer? How do you fix it? Don't worry, we'll get there! But the answer isn't so simple . . . because you're asking the wrong *question*. Let's back up.

Remember a time when sleep wasn't a big project? When it easily came most of the time, so much so that you didn't really think about it? Or maybe you've never had "easy" sleep, but you know this fabled thing exists because you've seen others simply lie down and take a nap like it was nothing, or listened to someone sleep like a log night after night (possibly while you pettily contemplated elbowing them awake just to show them what it's like).

So, when did you lose touch with sleep? When did it stop being an enjoyable thing and become a struggle instead? Take a pause and see if you can pinpoint where things started to go off track.

The evolution of your relationship with sleep might just mirror the way we, as a society, had our big falling out with it. In preindustrial times, we used to enjoy sleep as a natural experience—no user manual required—like breathing or lovemaking. We would sleep when the mood struck us, and just as simply, get up with the sun and the roosters, our natural alarm clocks. Sleep was a social experience, an opportunity to bond, rather than a private, slightly embarrassing biological necessity.

We held napping to be almost sacred. And as historian Roger Ekirch describes in "Sleep We Have Lost: Pre-Industrial Slumber in the British Isles,"* we thought there was nothing strange about waking up at 2:00 A.M. to do chores or sing songs before going back to bed for a "second sleep." We simply didn't have to work hard at it. There was a rhythm and a feeling . . . and we instinctively knew the how and when.

But then somebody invented artificial lights. Then came twenty-four-hour factories. Then a globalized economy. Industrialism and capitalism turned most people's bodies into tools for production, and along with this, our biological and psychological rhythms had to be wrangled into shape so they could serve as gears in "the machine."

Along the way, we lost some instincts, like our innate knowledge of where north lies, and our innate knowledge of how and when to sleep. Historian Benjamin Reiss describes in his book *Wild Nights: How Taming Sleep Created Our Restless World*† how during the rise of industrialization, Europeans began to get the sense that sleep was broken for "civilized" people (a.k.a., white Europeans). Medical writers blamed the rise in the prevalence of insomnia on the advancement of civilization and the "nerves" that come with superior intellect. Ironically, as Reiss documents, Europeans imperialized their brand of sleep at the same time—for example, teaching "savages" (a.k.a., the people they were colonizing) to sleep privately instead of socially. This is how, weirdly, sleep also took on a moral and political dimension. Perhaps that's why we still talk about sleep "hygiene," as if judging those who don't sleep in a specific way as being unclean or uncivilized.

At this point, it might seem like the answer is simple: Turn back the clock to that time of primeval sleep paradise. Just nap every day, throw

---

* Roger A. Ekirch, "Sleep we have Lost: Pre-Industrial Slumber in the British Isles," *The American Historical Review* 106, no. 2 (2001): 343–86.

† B. Reiss, *Wild Nights: How Taming Sleep Created our Restless World* (New York: Basic Books, 2017).

away screens, don't work so much, and tell your kids stories by candle-light.

Unfortunately, it's too late for that. This book is not about how we can restore good sleep by doing a Paleo sleep diet of never using artificial lights after sunset. Not only is that totally unfeasible, but it's also not the crux of the problem anymore. Our societal relationship with sleep continued to evolve, just as your personal relationship with sleep evolved over months or years, and now your sleeplessness isn't just about light, or stress, or disrupted biorhythms.

Insomnia has taken on a life of its own.

Now it's also the way we *think* about sleep and *act* around sleep that keeps the wedge between us and sleep. Every way you look, there is a new headline about how sleep deprivation will kill you or give you dementia (we'll talk about why that's misleading for people with insomnia in chapters 1 and 14), or how some new gadget will give you "advanced insights" for optimizing your sleep, or how these fifty-two tips will make you fall asleep in under five minutes. These threats and promises banish sleep to a cold and respectable distance, so we can turn our cold and objective gaze toward solving it as an engineering problem.

And maybe that's why business has never been better for the sleep industrial complex. Mattresses represent a $30 billion industry. Start-up companies promising *the* new sleep solution are getting more and more attention from Silicon Valley investors. The sleep aid market was worth $81.2 billion in 2020 and is projected to reach $112.7 billion in 2025.*

But as these technologies continue to advance at breakneck speed, are we getting any closer to our instinctive ability to sleep well? Now, instead of following our gut feelings, we try to coerce sleep into shape. But have you ever wondered: How did we manage before we had sleep tracking

---

* Business Communications Company, Inc. "Sleep Aids Market Size, Share & Industry Growth Analysis Report." Market Research Reports. 2021. https://www.bccresearch.com/market-research/healthcare/sleep-aids-techs-markets-report.html.

apps, Ambien, sleep music machines, $250 weighted blankets, lavender diffusers, and special mattresses that seem like greater feats of engineering than the Egyptian pyramids?

In short, something that used to be free, easy, and pleasurable has become one of society's most urgent and expensive problems. Somehow, our *relationship* with sleep has turned upside down.

Perhaps years ago, sleep was your intimate friend whose company you enjoyed, who brought you comfort instead of stress, and whose quirks you knew well and lovingly accepted. Now it's an old car that you use to get from point A to point B. You complain when it doesn't run smoothly. You buy tools and read mechanics' manuals to try to fix it. You take it to an expert for it to be prodded and treated.

What a sad turn of events! You've lost a friend and gained an engineering problem. And this is the same engineering problem Kate was trying to solve. Through sheer intellectual brute force, she tried to "hack" her own sleep. Somewhere in her data she thought she would find the algorithm to get her sleep back under her control.

But she was learning the hard way that sleep cannot be *controlled*. Just as you can't fake sexual desire or curb genuine surprise, you can't simply turn the dials on sleep. There are no dials. Sleep is too complex and—hopefully you'll agree by the end of this book—too beautiful for that. Scientists have been studying it for centuries and we still don't *really* understand what it is, much less precisely how it works.

Most basic sleep research is just a catalog of findings that made scientists go, "Whoa! Isn't that wild?" For example, did you know that our brains have little bursts of deep sleep while we're awake, and you can actually watch those undulating brain waves travel across the brain's surface the way water ripples across a pond (see chapter 1)? Did you know that little glitches in the transition from rapid eye movement (REM) sleep to wakefulness have given rise to demon mythologies and alien abduction conspiracies (see chapter 16)? Even without sophisticated scientific study, we can see that sleep is amazing. When else do we vividly hallucinate while our brains literally decide the fates of memories and massage our deepest emotions? I could gush all day about how cool sleep is.

"That's all well and good," you protest, "but how do I get more of all that goodness if I've lost control of my sleep?"

Remember: You can't control your sleep. This book will not teach you to do that. But here's the good news: you certainly don't *need* to control your sleep to have a lifelong, healthy relationship with it.

It might feel silly to use the term "relationship" here, as if sleep—a biological process—were a person with a mind of its own. But indulge me in this metaphor for a moment . . . Sleep, like a person, can indeed be unpredictable, stubborn, or even temperamental (otherwise you wouldn't have insomnia!). And sleep, like a person, does not like to be controlled. Bring to mind your best friend. Now imagine that you always dictate when and how long you spend time together, getting mad when she's not perfectly on your schedule. Imagine that you measure her "performance" every day, looking critically at her size and shape and blaming her when your day doesn't go well. Imagine that you won't give her space, instead keeping tabs on her all day and night, while also never appreciating that she does big favors for you all the time. Oh, and you never ask what *she* needs. Would your best friend still want to spend time with you? Now, why should sleep want to hang out with you if this is how you treat it?

You're not going to believe me right now, but here's the truth: You *do* know how to sleep, and how to do it well. What you need is not a formula to "fix" your sleep, because your sleep is not broken. What you need is not a collection of tips for how to "optimize" your sleep because perfection is neither necessary nor sufficient for sustainable sleep health.

What you need is to rebuild your friendship with sleep.

This means taking good care of your sleep but not being overbearing; it means having some meaningful boundaries but not letting rigid expectations rule the night; it means understanding what sleep needs from you instead of only what you want out of sleep. With this book I will help you by mediating this reconnection using the latest clinical sleep science. In part I, Get to Know Your Sleep, I'll guide you back to basics with a scientifically sound reintroduction to what healthy sleep looks like and what insomnia really means, so you can confidently navigate the Dr. Google headlines (spoiler: many of them are misleading!). You'll learn why sleep hygiene is used as the placebo condition in clinical trials for insomnia (spoiler: it's because it doesn't help insomnia), and what sleep specialists recommend instead.

In part II, we hit the Big Reset, reverting your sleep physiology and biological clock back to primal settings so you can begin a healthy relationship with sleep afresh. From there, we go deeper into the ways we think and act around sleep in part III, Going Deeper into the Relationship, learning to become experts in our own unhelpful patterns. In these two sections (II and III), which make up the "core" of the Hello Sleep program, I'll provide you with tools for understanding the sleep that is bespoke to *you*, not the standard-issue eight-hour mold. You'll learn practical how-tos for rebuilding a good relationship with your sleep, so you can not only fall asleep and stay asleep more easily but also feel better during the day.

For extra tailoring, part IV will answer your burning questions about changes in sleep as we age, women's sleep concerns (during pregnancy, postpartum, and menopause), special considerations when you have other medical/psychiatric disorders, and when to worry about other sleep disorders.

All these concepts and methods are based on cutting-edge sleep science, behavioral sleep medicine, and circadian science (i.e., how your biological clock works). We will especially lean on the most effective insomnia treatment in existence—cognitive behavioral therapy for insomnia (CBT-I), which the American College of Physicians has long stamped as the first-line treatment for any adult with insomnia. As a board-certified behavioral sleep medicine specialist, I can attest to the power of CBT-I, an approach I've used with countless patients who started out believing their sleep was broken and ended up with a new life. (By the way, if you think you've already tried CBT-I and it didn't work . . . read on, because not every provider delivers CBT-I the same way, and I bet there are important elements you haven't tried yet.)

But this book isn't just a step-by-step manual for putting yourself through CBT-I, a treatment that, in my opinion, can sometimes be too formulaic when you're not working one-on-one with an experienced specialist. (And those are hard to come by unless you live in San Francisco and have no problem with paying $300 out of pocket per forty-five-minute session). I'm a firm believer that people won't experience lasting change unless they reach a true understanding of the hows and whys.

That's why, instead of structuring this book to follow a standard progression of treatment sessions, I've organized it as a series of answers to questions you probably have about insomnia. You are welcome to browse or jump around the chapters at any pace, the way you'd enjoy a science book about jellyfish or the solar system. **If you want to use this book as a structured guide to overcome insomnia, I recommend reading the chapters in order. Dedicate six to ten weeks to work through the Hello Sleep program (parts II and III of this book), allocating about one full week to fully understand and implement the foundational concepts/skills for each chapter before moving on to the next.** The chapters in part IV are more like "a la carte" information you can browse at any time.

You can't change insomnia by only reading a book, just like you won't make friends by only reading a friendship manual. Even if you've fully grasped the concepts on an intellectual level, only the act of working through the exercises will change your relationship with sleep. So, do give the homework an honest shot, and I'll try to provide some guidance for when you can expect to see change. I always feel so bad when people give up on a foundational skill right before it starts to pay off for them!

Just a little spoiler here—Kate had a faltering start with sleep therapy, but she ended up doing beautifully. And it took less time than you might have guessed. From start to finish, I saw Kate five times, with sessions spaced one to two weeks apart. By the end, she had dropped her tug-of-war with sleep. She was no longer held hostage by the idea of controlling it. She was surprised at how well she could sleep, night after night, and how good she could feel during the day. And perhaps just as important, Kate didn't fret about sleep anymore, and instead, felt warmly toward her nightly companion. She and sleep were bosom friends again.

If Kate could fall in love with sleep, so can you. And when that happens, you'll have yourself a loyal companion for life, and you'll be experiencing sleep the way it's meant to be experienced—relaxing, gentle, and sweet.

PART I

Get to Know Your Sleep

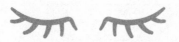

1

What Does Healthy Sleep Look Like?

You know that feeling of quiet bliss as you drift into sleep? That moment of tranquility where you are poised over the realm of sweet oblivion? How about that delicious feeling of waking up refreshed, like you've just slipped into the pool on a hot summer day?

Perhaps those are cruel questions. Since you're reading this book, experiences of tranquil sleep might be a distant memory, so obliterated by nights of struggling with insomnia that you hardly believe they ever existed. Or maybe you've always been a "bad sleeper," and this fabled experience of enjoying sleep is the unicorn you've chased for years. Perhaps your sleep isn't so bad, but you can't help but wonder if it couldn't be—or shouldn't be—better. Maybe if you slept eight to ten hours every night like Usain Bolt does, you'd be the fastest man on Earth . . . or at least have started training for that 5K. Or maybe you wonder if there are sleep hacks that, if deployed perfectly, could make you smarter, sexier, funnier, and all around more "optimized" as a human.

Whether you're desperate for a sleep cure or simply sleep curious,

I bet you've googled things like, "How much sleep do I need?" "What temperature is optimal for sleep?" "Tricks for falling asleep in 5 minutes." "Hacks for getting better sleep." But the answer to better sleep does not lie in the tips and tricks that you crave. Instead, it lies in the radical, but simple, idea that **healthy sleep comes from having a good relationship with sleep.** This means having an accurate understanding of how sleep works, both scientifically and experientially; knowing what you need to do to help your sleep thrive, and just as important, what you need to *refrain* from doing so as not to cramp its style. This means having appreciation and trust for your body's natural ability to sleep well, and being able to adapt with your sleep through the inevitable trials and tribulations of life.

This book will teach you how to do these things. It is meant for people who struggle with their sleep—those who can't turn off their brain when they go to bed at night, who stare at the ceiling (or their snoring spouse) with spite, who carry bricks of fatigue throughout their day, who worry that their sleeplessness will break down their body and mind, who crave rest that actually feels restful. I see you. I feel your struggle— that exhausting back-and-forth between hopelessness and desperation for satisfying sleep. And I have good news for you.

Insomnia is treatable. As a clinician with a short attention span and an almost pathologically strong sense of empathy, the only type of treatment I can do day in and day out is treatment that works (and works quickly). That's why, after my clinical psychology PhD training at Boston University, I chose to specialize in behavioral sleep medicine during my medical psychology residency and postdoctoral fellowship at the Duke University School of Medicine. Now, as a sleep researcher and clinician certified by the American Board of Behavioral Sleep Medicine, I spend most of my time helping people overcome insomnia. I am deeply gratified by helping patients go from "I've lost my ability to sleep" to "I can't believe it, but I'm a good sleeper" within a matter of weeks. I enjoy instilling hope for those who have been fighting a lonely battle for years. For delivering results using nothing more magical than scientifically based methods for resetting their sleep physiology and way of talking to themselves about sleep.

I wrote this book because people were asking me on Twitter about insomnia all the time, and my passionate responses never could fit within 280 characters. I wanted to write an up-to-date, laser-focused book on insomnia that was not simply a "layman's version" of sleep textbooks, but rather a fireside chat that treated my readers as intelligent, curious people capable of self-determination. I wanted to provide them with explanations that made sense and actually addressed their questions about insomnia—a collection of the scientifically sound but down-to-earth things I would say to my patients. So, I set out to write this book with the hope that people with insomnia will find within it the answers to their burning questions, and a practical plan to help them rekindle their love affair with sleep.

Let's get started.

To rebuild a good relationship with sleep, we have to get to know it. Like an old friend that you've drifted away from, what you think you know about sleep might not be true, or at least not true anymore. So, let's start with a blank slate. You've got a wide-open mind, and you're ready to get to know this wonderful thing called "sleep" from scratch.

What Is Sleep?

You would think that sleep is easily defined. But like jazz, it's actually hard to pin down a definition beyond, "You'll know it when you experience it." Scientists are still working on understanding exactly what it is, how it works, and why it happens. But so far, here's what we know with confidence:

- Sleep happens naturally, usually at more-or-less regular intervals.
- When we're asleep, we're less responsive to our surroundings than when we're awake, but more responsive than if we were in a coma.
- Brain activity is different during sleep compared to during wakefulness.
- When we don't sleep well for a long time, we feel bad, or our health or functioning may be negatively affected.

What Isn't Sleep?

- Sleep isn't your brain or body "shutting off." As you'll see, it's an active and dynamic state.
- Sleep isn't a skill you can (or need to) learn through hard work. It's an involuntary state that sometimes happens to you, and you can welcome it or allow it, but you can't summon it or control it.
- Sleep isn't the solution to all your problems. Expecting so will disappoint you and strain your sleep.

What Happens During Sleep?

The body and brain do some truly amazing things during sleep. Some of these include:

- Clearing out toxins from the cerebrospinal fluid (your brain "juices")
- Releasing human growth hormone and sex hormones

- Repairing damaged tissue and maintaining healthy tissue
- Reviewing and organizing new information
- Regulating emotions
- Practicing new skills

Notice that I didn't say, "Sleep does amazing things *for us.*" This is an important hair to split, because we shouldn't be treating sleep as a performance enhancer or tool. When we do, we unfairly put a lot of pressure on sleep to perform. Instead, consider sleep to simply be the enjoyable byproduct of these biological activities. In other words, sleep is neither our master nor servant, neither the answer to our problems nor the blame for them. It's hard to switch to this mindset, especially if you've been struggling with insomnia for a while, so be patient with yourself! Just start to notice whether you ever expect sleep to serve you (e.g., "I need to sleep so I can do well at my interview tomorrow"), and put a pin in this data point to examine later when you read part III, Getting Deeper into the Relationship.

The body and brain processes mentioned above take place during a few different types of sleep (sometimes referred to as "stages") that tend to tag-team in a pattern throughout the night. I'm not a fan of referring to types of sleep as "stages," because it's not like we're working through levels of a video game, where the goal is to go as far as possible, and you have to start over if you don't reach your objective. Not at all! It's more like sampling at a buffet, with second, third, and more helpings: alpha waves to start, then some spindles with K-complexes on the side, maybe some slow waves now (or REM, depending on what the brain's in the mood for), and then some more spindles to cleanse the palate. Yum! That's why I don't like to call different types of sleep "light" or "deep"; they imply "worse" or "better," whereas a good night of sleep needs all the different types of sleep (and wake), the same way a good meal needs a balance of vegetables, protein, and grains. Unfortunately, official sleep science terminology includes "stages," so that's what I'll use here to minimize confusion.

Stage 1 (Restful Wake)

Stage 1 is considered the lightest type of sleep because we are easily woken from it, and during it, we may not feel like we're sleeping at all. That's why it's sometimes called "restful wake." It takes up only about 5 percent of a typical night, serving mostly as a transition between waking and other types of sleep.

Stage 2 (Light Sleep)

Even though Stage 2 is considered "light sleep," it is actually an active and important time for the brain. This stage produces electrical activity bursts called spindles, which help our brains to cement new learning. There are also K-complexes, a twitch in the electroencephalogram (EEG) waveform we don't fully understand, which might reflect a moment where the brain scans the environment for new inputs. When you learn new things during the day, whether it's French verb conjugations or how to serve a tennis ball, your brain fires up sleep spindles during Stage 2, and you wake up with more mastery of the skill than you had when you went to bed. This type of sleep takes up approximately 45 percent to 55 percent of the night. Yes, you read that correctly . . . **fully half the night is supposed to be spent in this "light" stage of sleep**, and it's time well-spent!

Stage 3 (Slow Wave Sleep, Deep Sleep)

This type of sleep is called "slow wave sleep" because the brain activity you see on an EEG looks like big, rolling waves, unlike the usually tight, frenetic smaller waves we have when awake or in other types of sleep. During Stage

3, the brain's lymphatic system does important janitorial work to clear toxins from the brain. It also releases growth and sex hormones, helps us to cement new learning, and engages in general rest and restoration . . . all nice things. People usually refer to Stage 3 as "deep sleep," but please don't think this means it's the only good type of sleep, or that it's better than the others—this is a common myth! **In fact, Stage 3 sleep is only supposed to take up about 15 percent to 20 percent of a typical night for a healthy adult sleeper, and even less if they're past middle age.** This type of sleep mostly happens during the first half of your night.

Rapid Eye Movement Sleep

Rapid eye movement, or REM, sleep is very different from the other three (those are collectively known as "non-REM" stages). During REM, your major muscles are deactivated, your eyes move behind closed lids, and your brain's EEG pattern looks almost like when awake. The brain is very active—it sorts through memories, makes sense of emotions, makes decisions about what to keep and what to lose. Think of a detective sorting through their wall of interlinked mug shots and news clippings and question marks with an intense soundtrack playing in the background. With all this action, it's no surprise that REM is also when most of our dreaming happens.

Wake

Yes, if we're going to walk through a healthy, typical night of sleep, we're going to have to talk about wakefulness. **A healthy adult of about thirty-five to sixty-five years old wakes about ten to sixteen times per night**, though they don't remember most of these brief awakenings. (Older adults wake even more frequently.) It's normal to remember a few awakenings: going to the bathroom, adjusting your position, getting a sip of water, or being startled by a noise or dream. Don't worry about these events interrupting your sleep. (I repeat: do not worry.) Your brain naturally interrupts your sleep multiple times per hour anyway. A dozen or so brief awakenings (including a few that you remember, each lasting a few minutes) is totally normal, so don't get upset if your sleep tracker says you woke up ten or twenty times last night. Waking up briefly doesn't mean you're starting a sleep cycle over or missing out on a particular stage of sleep. An exception is if you have obstructive sleep apnea or other serious sleep disorders that wake you up every few minutes throughout the night (see chapter 16).

The Myth of Sleep "Cycles"

Our brains move through these types of sleep in a more or less predictable pattern, with some variations from night to night, person to person. This pattern is called *sleep architecture*. Just as I don't like the terminology of sleep "stages," I also don't like to refer to sleep architecture patterns as "sleep cycles." You may have heard that sleep cycles are ninety minutes long, and that you should try to time your wake-up alarm to be at the end of a cycle.

Nope. Forget that.

Sleep architecture doesn't follow a lather-rinse-repeat pattern because so-called sleep cycles are not that neat. Even your own "cycles" are not the same shape or length during one night, and sleep architecture doesn't look the same between you and me. Besides, the boundaries between the different "stages" of sleep are blurry. While one part of the brain is in Stage 2, another might have sidled on to REM.* While most of the brain is awake, a Stage 2 sleep spindle or two can pop up here and

---

* Joshua J. Emrick, Brooks A. Gross, Brett T. Riley, and Gina R. Poe, "Different Simultaneous Sleep States in the Hippocampus and Neocortex," *SLEEP* 39, no. 12 (2016): 2201–09. https://doi.org/10.5665/sleep.6326.

there, and even Stage 3 slow waves might roll in briefly.* During deep sleep, your brain isn't all slow wave electrical activity. These undulating waves travel from brain region to brain region, like a tornado sweeping across the landscape of your cortex, the wrinkly outer layer of your brain. So, to say that someone "cycles" through sleep stages is like saying the Rolling Stones cycle through chords. It oversimplifies a complex, mysterious, and beautiful phenomenon. And because sleep architecture is so wonderfully messy, we can't control it.

But don't worry—you don't need to control your sleep stages. **Your brain will automatically adjust how much deep sleep versus REM sleep versus light sleep you get, in what sequence, and in which brain regions, all dependent on your current needs.** This flexibility is a good thing! Some days you learn to serve a tennis ball and other days you watch emotional documentaries. Some days are long, and some are short. Your brain will know what to do with each type of sleep in each of these situations.

SOAPBOX MOMENT

Why is this "sleep cycle" idea so popular? I believe it's partly driven by our collective desire to control sleep with technology. We'll talk in detail about sleep gadgets in chapter 3, but for now, know this—you should trust your own brain before trusting a gadget that supposedly wakes you up at the "end of a cycle," because (1) current gadgets are not actually good at discerning sleep stages and (2) this concept is arbitrary and irrelevant . . . it's not like the sleep you get doesn't count unless you somehow stick the landing with a perfectly timed bout of REM.

---

* Yval Nir, Richard J. Staba, Thomas Andrillon, Vladyslav V. Vyazovskiy, Chiara Cirelli, Itzhak Fried, and Giulio Tononi, "Regional Slow Waves and Spindles in Human Sleep," *Neuron* 70, no.1 (2011): 153–69. https://doi.org/10.1016/j.neuron.2011.02.043.

What Is Healthy Sleep (and the Eight-Hour Myth)?

Healthy sleep simply happens when your brain and body do all the functions they need to meet their needs. Ideally, healthy sleep is also sleep that you feel good about.

But, of course, what most people mean when they ask this question is, "How much sleep do I need?" I'm sure you've heard that you should get eight hours of sleep per night. This is like Dr. Google saying that you need eight glasses of water per day. Does this apply to Megan Rapinoe during the height of soccer training season, or me (a petite couch potato) during a Netflix marathon? Should a construction worker in the Arizona desert drink the same amount of water as a librarian in rainy Seattle?

The same logic applies to sleep. **Not only do you and I differ in the amount (and timing) of sleep we need, we ourselves might change from day to day, week to week, season to season, and certainly over the course of our lives.** When pregnant, sleep changes. When training for a marathon, sleep changes. When going through a breakup, moving from the city to the country, coping with jet lag, starting a job, losing a job, recovering from the flu, learning to play the trumpet, going through puberty, retiring* . . . if you just saw your life flash before your eyes, close them and take a deep breath. Sleep changes a lot. This is *normal*. That's because sleep is stretchy and resilient by design. Why?

Envision a band of early humans trying to survive on the savannah. Imagine if everyone in the tribe dropped into an uninterrupted sleep at the exact same time for the exact same duration, every night. If I were a saber-toothed tiger, I'd just camp out near this hominid buffet and leisurely sharpen my claws all day. I'd know that this completely predictable species will serve up a completely defenseless dinner every night.

---

* There is even some new evidence that the phase of the moon is associated with how much and when people sleep.

Our prehistoric ancestors needed restless night owls, bright-eyed morning larks, light sleepers, dead logs, middle-of-the-night risers, middle-of-the-day nappers, and sleepers of all sorts. This diversity saved lives and perpetuated our species. They needed wise elders who needed less sleep to watch over exhausted hunters, who probably needed more; they needed morning birds to get the bows strung bright and early, as well as night owls to keep an eye out for predators of the night.* In summer, they needed to be stimulated by sunlight so they could hunt and gather, and in winter they needed to save energy because there wasn't much hunting or gathering to do. When there was danger on the horizon, they needed to turn from sleepy to alert on a dime, but also to conserve energy when food was scarce.

This is why evolution made our sleep so diverse and dynamic. And this is why LeBron James sleeps twelve hours per night and Terry Gross probably doesn't (unless she has a secret life as a professional weightlifter in addition to hosting the radio talk show *Fresh Air*).

Even if we had to boil the complex question of optimal sleep duration down to simple headlines, "eight hours" still wouldn't be the best answer. For example, a recent large study of older Japanese adults found that those sleeping, on average, between five and seven hours per night had the lowest rate of death and dementia over time, compared to those who slept less or more.† You might have guessed that less than five hours of sleep per night is not ideal, but perhaps you hadn't considered that longer sleep durations can be associated with health problems too. In fact, in the most recent meta-analysis‡ on the topic, data from more

---

* Disclaimer: All the evolutionary stuff I talk about here is educated speculation based on principles, such as "Diversity is generally good for a species' survival." I don't have actual footage of prehistoric hominids doing night-shift security work.

† Tomoyuki Ohara, Takanori Honda, Jun Hata, Daigo Yoshida, Naoko Mukai, Yoichiro Hirakawa, Mao Shibata, et al., "Association Between Daily Sleep Duration and Risk of Dementia and Mortality in a Japanese Community," *Journal of the American Geriatrics Society* 66, no. 10 (2018): 1911–18. https://doi.org/10.1111/jgs.15446.

‡ A meta-analysis is a type of study that pools data from a bunch of studies, making its conclusions the most trustworthy.

than forty-three thousand participants tracked over time showed that long sleep duration (eight hours per night or more) was linked to a 77 percent increased risk for dementia, whereas short sleep duration (less than six hours per night) was not associated with increased risk for dementia.* I am not recommending that you prevent yourself from ever getting more than six hours of sleep per night. As we'll see below, these types of studies don't tell us the optimal amount of sleep for each of us.

So how come different studies seem to come up with different numbers? First, there's no perfect agreement between researchers about what "short sleep" means,† so we group hundreds or thousands of participants into this category, including ones who sleep less than five hours, but sometimes also including ones who sleep seven or eight hours, depending on where a particular research team decides to draw the line. When data are pooled together like this, it's impossible to tell if it's the five-hour sleepers or the seven-hour sleepers in the "short sleeper" group that are driving the results.

Second, researchers measure sleep differently. Some of these studies base their sleep duration analyses on a single questionnaire item asking, "Approximately how many hours do you sleep per night?" Other studies ask participants to painstakingly track their sleep for many nights using multiple tools, or measure their sleep using sophisticated equipment in the lab. It's safe to assume that almost all headlines refer to ballparks and guesstimates.

Last, but not least, these different studies included different samples of people. Some followed young adults, others older adults; some

---

* Li Fan, Weihao Xu, Yulun Cai, Yixin Hu, and Chenkai Wu, "Sleep Duration and the Risk of Dementia: A Systematic Review and Meta-Analysis of Prospective Cohort Studies," *Journal of the American Medical Directors Association* 20, no. 12 (2019): 1480–1487. https://doi.org/10.1016/j.jamda.2019.06.009.

† Lisa Gallicchio, and Bindu Kalesan, "Sleep Duration and Mortality: A Systematic Review and Meta-Analysis," *Journal of Sleep Research* 18, no. 2 (2009): 148–58. https://doi.org/10.1111/j.1365-2869.2008.00732.x.

followed people at risk for disease, while others followed only healthy people; some studies were done in the United States, others in Japan, the Netherlands, Turkey, or elsewhere. By now, you've gathered that headlines don't tell the whole story, and that things can get quite messy when we dig into details.

One thing that pretty much all large-scale studies about sleep duration agree on: long sleep duration, *usually* defined as more than nine or ten hours per night, is associated with more health problems over time.

Does this mean you should never let yourself sleep more than nine hours? Or place any other specific limit or expectation on your nightly sleep duration? The answer is no. Here's why:

- **Correlation is not causation**. Just because people who sleep nine hours per night are statistically more likely to also have dementia doesn't mean it's the long sleep that *causes* dementia. Maybe it's the other way around—having brain changes related to dementia causes someone to become sleepier. Or maybe both things are caused by a whole other factor. **If your body tells you that you need nine hours of sleep, there's no need to deprive yourself.** But if it's your *thoughts* that tell you you need a specific amount of sleep or else you'll die young . . . we have some work to do in part III of this book.
- Someone who averages, say, seven hours per night sometimes sleeps more than that, and sometimes less . . . **you're allowed to have fluctuations**.
- The problem with talking about *averages* is that **you may not be average.***
- Even if you are average for your demographic, **the type and**

---

* Another problem with averages is that sometimes they don't make sense. My husband and I have, on average, one testicle each. Not a particularly useful statistic.

amount of sleep you need may not match the average for the people in any particular study. For example, most of you are probably not Japanese sixty-seven-year-olds.

- It comes down to this: **There is no single correct way to sleep. Many shapes and sizes of sleep are healthy if they answer your body's needs at this time in your life.**

So Why Does the National Sleep Foundation (and My Doctor) Say I Should Get Seven to Nine Hours of Sleep per Night?

If you dig beneath the headlines, you'll find that the National Sleep Foundation actually believes that anywhere between five and eleven hours "may be appropriate" for adults.* That's why it took this entire chapter to tell you about healthy sleep. It can't be boiled down to just a couple of numbers.

Also, I think there is always some tension between public health messaging and individual health advice. There are likely more people who don't give themselves enough *opportunity* to sleep (e.g., college students pulling all-nighters, professionals who are married to their email) than people who have chronic insomnia. So, a reasonable public health message, if it needs to fit in a headline, may err on the side of recommending more sleep than many people need (eight hours per night). But this is at the expense of many people with insomnia, especially older adults who are conscientious about sleep but simply don't need eight hours.

---

* Max Hirshkowitz, Kaitlyn Whiton, Steven M. Albert, Cathy Alessi, Oliviero Bruni, Lydia DonCarlos, Nancy Hazen, et al., "National Sleep Foundation's Sleep Time Duration Recommendations: Methodology and Results Summary," *Sleep Health: Journal of the National Sleep Foundation* 1, no. 1 (2015): 40–43. https://doi.org/10.1016/J.SLEH.2014.12.010.

It's Not Just About the Nighttime Either

So far we've talked about what happens at night. But talking only about nighttime sleep is like talking only about waves while ignoring the tide. Sleep doesn't happen in a vacuum. It's part of a larger system of rhythms in our bodies that are called *circadian rhythms*. The Latin words *circa* and *dian* mean "about a day," so circadian rhythms simply refer to "approximately daily rhythms." They can be found in the daily fluctuations of our core body temperature, hormone levels, metabolic function, attention span, mood . . . every experience we have ebbs and flows in rhythm as part of this tide, this circadian system.

Why is the circadian system important for sleep? Years ago, I got to watch the Boston Symphony Orchestra rehearse (actual performances were too expensive for a grad student!). Some performances really took my breath away. Even aside from the artistry of the music, it always amazed me that a hundred separate instruments being played by a hundred different musicians could all come together as a single organism to create this perfect, precise piece of music.

In a way, our bodies are like orchestras. Our billions of cells, most with their own circadian clocks, come together as tissues and organs and organ systems that all must "play" in sync to keep us functioning. And like an orchestra, there is someone conducting the show—the suprachiasmatic nucleus (SCN). The SCN, which I think is the most underrated brain nucleus, is a tiny, pea-sized region deep in the brain that acts as your circadian system's maestro. This "maestro" needs to keep a billion-member "orchestra" perfectly on time and in sync. When it knows what time it is, it can do its job well, and the orchestra hits every note beautifully. Your body and brain will know what to do and when to do it, including when to be sleepy and when to be awake. But if the maestro is confused, perhaps because you have no consistent schedule from day to day, they will not be able to lead the orchestra well. In that case, everything—including your sleep and wake—will suffer.

What Is the Best Time to Sleep? (Know Your Chronotype)

So how can we keep our maestro happy and our circadian system functioning well? As we'll see in part II, The Big Reset, day versus night contrast and day-to-day consistency are key. That means making it very easy for our brains to tell when it's daytime versus nighttime, and keeping stable patterns in what time of day our major biological activities occur—including when we sleep and when we wake.

Many patients then ask, "What is the best time to sleep, then? I heard that we get our best sleep from X o'clock to Y o'clock." But just as we're all different in how *much* sleep we need, we also differ in *when* we naturally want to sleep. This also changes over a lifetime, which parents know because their five-year-old used to come crashing into their bed at 6:00 A.M. and now, ten years later, the same kid doesn't get up until noon. You may remember how, in college, you had plenty of energy past midnight, whether it was for studying or partying, but now you can't keep your eyes open past 10:30 P.M. By the time you're eighty years old, you may drift off even earlier in the evening, and be up before dawn with no alarm needed.

These tendencies in when we want to sleep versus when we feel alert are called chronotypes. You may have heard of night owls (people who tend to sleep later and wake later) and morning larks (those who sleep early and wake early). You may even have taken an online quiz about what your "sleep animal" is, which is loosely meant to tell you what chronotype you have. But really, everybody just falls somewhere along a continuum, just as our heights fall on a continuum.

I want to emphasize that there is nothing inherently good or bad, healthy or unhealthy, about any chronotype. We tend to stigmatize

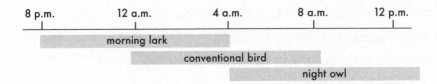

night owls by calling them "lazy" or saying they *should* get up at a "decent" hour. The truth is, you can be lazy or productive no matter what your chronotype is.

Although there is research showing that people with later chronotypes (i.e., night owls) are more prone to depression,* this is because they're having to bend their natural chronotype to societal norms, which are designed for morning people. The problem isn't with their natural chronotype, but rather with the fact that they don't get enough sleep because they have to get up earlier than desired to catch that 8:00 A.M. class, or because they are switching between 6:00 A.M. weekday wakeups and 9:00 A.M. weekend wakeups, jet lagging themselves from New York to Los Angeles and back every week. If they were simply allowed to sleep during their natural chronotype window, let's say 2:00 A.M. to 10:00 A.M., they would be perfectly happy, healthy, and productive.

We'll discuss chronotypes and circadian rhythms in more detail in chapters 6 and 16. For now, start asking yourself what your natural chronotype may be. Do you feel most energetic and productive in the morning or the evening? If you were on vacation with no obligations whatsoever and nobody (including yourself) to judge you, when would you naturally sleep and wake? When in your life did you feel best about your sleep-wake schedule, and when were you getting up in those days?

Remember that working *with* your body, instead of *against*, is always easier and healthier. If you have the luxury of flexibility in your

---

* J. Au and J. Reece, "The Relationship Between Chronotype and Depressive Symptoms: A Meta-analysis," *Journal of Affective Disorders*, 218 (2017), 93–104.

daytime obligations, don't arbitrarily pick a time to get up just because that's when ultra-productive tech CEOs claim to be getting up. Don't arbitrarily pick a time to go to bed just because it's a "decent" hour to do so. Listen to your own body.

How Can We Get Healthy Sleep?

So, it seems like the only "rule" so far is that everybody is different, and everybody changes over time. How are we supposed to get the right amount of sleep at the right times if we don't know all the variables in the algorithm, and even the ones we know, we often can't control?

That was a trick question. Ask a good sleeper, "How do you do it?" Their answer is likely to be, "I don't know. I just sleep."

Don't get mad. They're not selfishly withholding their secret to good sleep. They're not trying to brag about how such a difficult task is so easy for them. They honestly don't know how they sleep so well! And that's because they don't actually *do* anything about their sleep. In fact, they probably don't think much about their sleep at all.

The good news is that, once we have a good relationship with sleep, we don't have to consciously calculate, control, manage, plan, strategize, or hack anything either. The brain will do all the calculations behind the scenes, and your only job is to enjoy the experience, the same way your infuriatingly good sleeper of a coworker simply enjoys the experience. To get to this point in your relationship, all you have to do is:

1. Learn to listen to your body.
2. Learn what behaviors and attitudes are getting in the way of your good sleep.

The rest of this book is all about how to do these two things. To become good at the first one, you can start by letting go of the idea that you know or can figure out exactly how much sleep you need. Sometimes this stubborn idea disguises itself in the form of, "If only I could get half an hour more per night, I'd be golden" or "I'm not asking for eight hours per night, but shouldn't I get at least X hours?"

Instead, I invite you to start feeling instead of thinking. Specifically, feel what "sleepy" feels like. Ask yourself, with genuine curiosity, "What does it feel like in my body when I get sleepy versus when I get tired? How do I know which one I'm feeling? How do my eyes feel? My head, hands, legs?" No need to change anything or try to create any feelings. Just ride along with whatever comes up.

This may not feel like you're doing much, but that's the point. **Know that by simply switching from a *doing* mode to *noticing* mode, you have started your journey to restoring a healthy relationship with sleep!** After all, in couples counseling, isn't the first step to simply listen to each other?

In the next chapter we'll dig into what exactly insomnia is, and more important, what it *isn't*. We'll also walk through the steps of how you developed insomnia, which will help you to begin mapping a path out of its shadow.

BOTTOM LINE

- Healthy sleep is diverse and dynamic. It's different between you and me. Even within the same person, it changes from day to day, week to week, and year to year.
- There are different types of sleep (often called "stages"), all of which are good and important. The brain samples them in a somewhat predictable pattern over the course of a night, but it also adjusts the size and shape of your sleep architecture depending on your needs at the moment. Usually, a healthy sleeper only needs 15 percent to 20 percent of their night to be "deep" sleep.

- Studies show that there is a range for how much sleep could be optimal, but that eight hours is probably not the best answer for many adults. The only way to know your current "optimal" is to learn to listen to your body (and get out of its way).
- The timing of our sleep and wake is just as important as how *much* sleep we're getting. This, too, differs between people and changes across the lifetime. Get to know your chronotype so you can work *with*, instead of *against*, your body.
- To achieve your own healthy sleep, you can begin by learning to switch from *doing* to *noticing* mode. This means noticing what "sleepy" feels like in your body, without judgment or effort. This is your first piece of homework.

What Is Insomnia and How Did I Get It?

K ate is a successful data scientist. She and her husband are parents of twin seven-year-old boys. Kate used to be someone people described as "full of life." She's still generally healthy and upbeat, but for the past few years everything seems weighed down by her nocturnal struggles. Kate dreads going to bed every night, because she knows she will toss and turn, sometimes for hours, trying to shut down her racing mind. Even after she falls asleep, she wakes up repeatedly and watches the angry red numbers on her alarm clock chart the course through every witching hour. She tries very hard not to take Lunesta, but sometimes the 2:00 A.M. desperation leaves her no choice. Some mornings, an exhausted Kate lets herself cry for a couple of minutes in the kitchen before the rest of the family wakes up, already feeling defeated about making it through the day on so little sleep.

What Is Insomnia?

You don't need to go to medical school to know what insomnia is. It's simply when a person has serious trouble with falling or staying asleep.

This happens to pretty much everybody at least sometimes—on nights before having to catch an early flight, on nights after having a fight with their partner, on the night before an interview or wedding or trip to Disney World . . . that's totally normal and okay.

Insomnia disorder, or *chronic* insomnia, is more of a problem. This is when we're no longer just talking about a few nights of sleep struggles once in a while. Chronic insomnia is diagnosed when*

- there's trouble with falling and/or staying asleep on about half the nights or more;
- it's been happening for longer than a couple of months;
- it's causing problems with mood, functioning, energy, or well-being during the day;
- there's not a very obvious external reason for the sleep problem, such as drinking a lot of coffee in the evening, having to caretake or respond to crises at night, having a foghorn that blows right outside the bedroom window, etc.; and
- there's not another medical, psychiatric, or sleep disorder that explains the insomnia; if this other condition were cured, the insomnia would likely still stick around.

But knowing what insomnia *isn't* is just as important as knowing what it *is*, because we don't want to be chasing the wrong leads. So, let's set the record straight on some common misconceptions about insomnia.

Insomnia Is Not Failing to Meet a Specific Sleep Quota

You probably noticed from the diagnostic criteria for insomnia disorder that **there are no specific cutoffs for how much sleep or wakefulness**

---

* American Psychiatric Association, *Diagnostic and Statistical Manual-5th Edition* (American Psychiatric Association Publishing: 2013), 362–368. https://doi.org/10.1176/appi.books.9780890425596.744053.

constitutes insomnia. "Difficulty falling and/or staying asleep" is intentionally vague, because insomnia doesn't mean "less than X hours of sleep" or "taking longer than Y minutes to fall asleep" or "waking up Z number of times." Insomnia is mostly in the eye of the beholder. So, if taking ten minutes to fall asleep bothers you a lot and ruins your day, then ten minutes counts as "difficulty falling asleep." If you're happy with taking sixty minutes from lights out to sleeping and it's not causing you problems, you do *not* have "difficulty falling asleep."

Insomnia Is Not Just a Nighttime Problem

I'm betting that insomnia doesn't just bother you at night. I'm sure it's something you fret about during the day (understandably), something that takes up mental space and emotional bandwidth. Like Kate, you may even dread the thought of it leading up to bedtime or change your evening plans according to how much sleep problems you anticipate. Insomnia also makes you feel lousy—you're tired, foggy, irritable, and dogged by a feeling that you could be so much happier and more productive if only you slept better.

Insomnia is a twenty-four-hour disorder. And the daytime component of insomnia is more than half of the puzzle. To overcome insomnia, almost all the changes you will need to make will happen when you're awake. (This is good news, since you have much more control over what you do when you're conscious!)

Insomnia Is Not Just a Symptom of Stress

Often, people are advised that if they learn to manage their stress better, they would not have insomnia anymore. This is frustrating to many people with years-long insomnia, because often they are not particularly stressed (except about the whole insomnia thing), or they are, but "self-care" and meditation haven't helped their sleep much. This is because chronic insomnia, even if initially triggered by a stressful period, is mostly maintained by other factors in the long term (see the section Perpetuating Factors near the end of this chapter). But surely my stressful and anxious thoughts are the things fueling my racing mind and keeping me awake! It can certainly feel like that, but guess what—if you were sleepy enough, your mind would have no opportunity to race. Don't worry, this will make more sense as you go through the Hello Sleep program.

Insomnia Is Not Due to a Chemical Imbalance in the Brain or Malfunctioning Brain Area

Well, it kind of is because our brain is involved in everything we experience and do. Even irritable bowel syndrome, for example, affects (and is affected by) the serotonin system in the brain. Similarly, the brain functions of people with insomnia versus without are somewhat different, reflecting differences in hyperarousal (a concept you'll become familiar with in part II of this book), but chronic insomnia is not *caused* by a breakdown of any brain structure or a shortage of some neurochemical in the way that, say, Parkinson's disease is a breakdown of the basal ganglia and a shortage of dopamine.* And we know this because insomnia *can* be resolved without taking neurochemical-altering medications or neurosurgery. You'll have to take my word for it, but as you begin to systematically change the barriers to your sleep, you'll see that the real culprits of insomnia are rather mundane and much more within your control than "chemical imbalance."

---

* This is an oversimplification of Parkinson's disease, of course. This disease is close to my heart because my doctoral dissertation was about its relationship with sleep and circadian rhythms. The generous people who volunteered to be in my study will forever have my gratitude.

COMMON MISCONCEPTION: INSOMNIA IS UNTREATABLE

There seems to be a common misconception, even among reputable scientists and doctors, that insomnia is due to mysterious and untreatable biological forces. Even highly respected sleep physicians who are experts at treating other sleep disorders (e.g., sleep apnea and narcolepsy) sometimes shrug about insomnia and tell people to simply accept that they'll have to live with it forever.

I cannot stress this enough: Insomnia is very treatable. Treating insomnia in all of its forms is the bread and butter of what we behavioral sleep medicine specialists do, and we do it quite successfully most of the time, because we *do* understand and address the biological (and other forces) that keep insomnia going. Unfortunately, the good news of behavioral insomnia treatment has not spread far and wide through the healthcare community, despite being the gold standard approach according to the American Academy of Sleep Medicine (AASM). There is nothing "alternative" about behavioral sleep medicine! So, don't be discouraged.

Insomnia Is Not Inevitable, Even If You and Your Whole Family Have Always Been Bad Sleepers

Many patients tell me that they were bad sleepers since they were babies. Many have parents who are "lifelong insomniacs." Understandably, they feel destined to a lifetime of bad sleep.

First, regarding babies and kids: Having a baby that doesn't sleep through the night is like having a lasagna that is delicious—totally expected. Children, too, can be "bad sleepers" through no fault of their genes (or parents, for that matter). They are designed to test boundaries and exploit parents' unconditional love, so it's not hard to get into patterns of repeated curtain calls at bedtime, or middle-of-the-night demands for comfort. Other sleep disruptors like sleepwalking, night terrors, and bedwetting are also common.

Teenagers are even more star-crossed when it comes to sleep. From their biological hardwiring as night owls clashing with ridiculously early school start times (I could go on about this) to social and academic pressures to exploding needs for independence . . . sleep is almost inevitably affected. I don't say all this to scare parents about how poorly their kids will sleep. I just want to reassure you that, **if you were a "bad sleeper" as a baby/child/teen, this by no means indicates some fundamental inability to sleep well**.

What if your parents had insomnia too? Could it be that it runs in your family? Don't worry, insomnia is not like Huntington's disease, where the genetic heritability is high and having a parent with the disease gives someone a coin flip's chance of having it too. Genes do play a part in insomnia—a recent genome-wide association study with more than 1.3 million participants found 202 gene loci that may have to do with insomnia, but all together, they only explained 7 percent of the phenotypic variance.* In English: Of all the reasons why you have insomnia while your brother (or daughter, friend, neighbor) doesn't, only a very small portion has to do with genes. This is good news again because nongenetic things are much easier to change.

Insomnia Is Not an Umbrella Term for a Big Variety of Disorders

Some websites (and outdated medical texts) will tell you that there are many types of insomnia: primary insomnia, secondary insomnia, sleep

---

* P. R. Jansen, K. Watanabe, S Stringer, N Skene, J. Bryois, A. R. Hammerschlag, et al., "Genome-wide Analysis of Insomnia in 1,331,010 Individuals Identifies New Risk Loci and Functional Pathways," *Nature genetics* 5, no. 3: 394–403.

onset insomnia, sleep maintenance insomnia, psychophysiological insomnia, paradoxical insomnia, idiopathic insomnia, insomnia due to [insert other problem], etc. Don't be intimidated by these seemingly complicated terms. We now know that they all essentially operate by the same principles.

For example, we used to distinguish between primary insomnia and secondary insomnia (the latter is now more accurately called comorbid insomnia). Primary insomnia is when someone only has insomnia and is in otherwise good health. Secondary insomnia, or comorbid insomnia, is when someone has insomnia as well as another significant health condition, such as cancer, chronic pain, depression, or other illnesses that can make sleep worse. Having a comorbid condition can certainly complicate sleep, but it doesn't make *chronic* insomnia inevitable. That's because chronic insomnia is not kept alive in the long run by pain or anxiety, even if it was triggered by them in the first place. Instead, it's kept alive by the way we respond to the disrupted sleep, which we *can* influence. This means comorbid insomnia can be improved with the same methods that improve primary insomnia, and doing so might even make the other condition better or easier to cope with.

Don't get caught up in what you've heard about different types of insomnia. It's not that complicated. The only types that matter are short term versus long term. I'm betting because you're reading this book, you've already been dealing with insomnia for more than a few weeks, so from here on, when I say "insomnia," I will be talking about long-term, or chronic, insomnia.

Insomnia Is Not Chronic Sleep Deprivation

I know, I know. This sounds crazy. Having insomnia means that you aren't getting enough sleep, right? But think of it this way: **If you are**

sleep-deprived, you would be very sleepy (and I mean *sleepy*, not tired),* just like if you were food-deprived, you would be very hungry. And if you were very sleepy, you would easily fall and stay asleep. If you can easily fall and stay asleep, by definition, you don't have insomnia.

Let me say that again: If someone deprived you of sleep the way war criminals torture prisoners, let's say by dousing you with cold water, playing startling sounds, or blasting you with pain every time you nod off, you would become sleepier and sleepier the longer you're forcibly kept awake. Eventually, you'd be so sleepy that you'd fall asleep standing on ice with a horn blowing in your ear. In other words, **sleep deprivation makes people sleepy**. If you have insomnia, your *inability* to sleep (in a bed, with no torture machines!) is direct proof that you are probably not sleep deprived.

There's further proof: In a classic research study,† ten people with insomnia (chronic trouble falling or staying asleep) were paired up with ten healthy sleepers who were otherwise very similar. The researchers first measured each insomniac's sleep overnight in the lab using the precise method of polysomnography, which involves monitoring brain waves, muscle activity, eye movements, heart rhythms, and other physiological activities. This multichannel ensemble produces a minute-by-minute readout of whether a person is asleep. Then, the researchers replicated the readouts, minute-by-minute, in the matched healthy sleeper partner—the partner was not allowed to fall asleep until the time the insomniac finally fell asleep, and whenever the insomniac was awake during the night, the partner would get woken up at the same time and for the same duration. They did this to the healthy sleepers for seven nights in a row. This essentially resulted in the healthy sleepers "walking

---

* This *sleepy* versus *tired* distinction is crucial to understanding insomnia. Tired = feeling worn out, depleted, exhausted, bored, low energy, etc. Sleepy = you're about to fall asleep. We'll continue to hammer this home.

† M. H. Bonnet and D. L. Arand, "The Consequences of a Week of Insomnia," *Sleep* 19, no. 6: 453–61.

a mile" in the insomniac's shoes for a whole week, having experienced close to the exact same sleep pattern and sleep amount. What would you guess happened to each person?

Let's start with the obvious. The healthy sleepers experienced symptoms of mild sleep deprivation, including:

- Decreased vigor
- Decreased tension
- Decreased body temperature
- Increased sleepiness*
- Underestimation of sleep problem (i.e., they were awake during the night longer than they realized)

Most of this is unsurprising—being woken up when you would otherwise be sleeping is sleep deprivation, and experiencing this repeatedly over a week would, of course, lead to some impairment. The only surprising thing was that they also experienced *decreased* tension—the mild sleep deprivation did not seem to bother them or rev them up.

The surprising part is what happened to the insomniacs. First, remember that the researchers didn't *do* anything to the insomniacs. They just slept as they usually did, insomnia and all. Whatever they experienced after a week of insomnia is just the natural consequence of having trouble falling/staying asleep even when nobody is purposefully keeping them awake. These consequences included:

- *Increased* tension
- *Increased* body temperature
- *Decreased* sleepiness

---

* In the lab, sleep researchers measure a person's level of sleepiness in a very simple way: How long does it take someone to fall asleep if they're put in a quiet, dark room and asked to take a nap? The less time it takes for them to fall asleep, the sleepier they are. This is called the multiple sleep latency test.

- *Overestimation* of sleep problem (i.e., they thought they had more trouble falling asleep than they actually did)
- No data on changes in vigor

Aside from not having information about vigor (too bad, because I'm curious!), notice that the outcomes in insomniacs are the exact *opposite* of what the healthy sleepers experienced after having the *same* sleep pattern. And here's a bonus finding: as closely as the researchers tried to match the pair's sleep patterns exactly, they couldn't control specific sleep stages, and although most sleep stage patterns were similar between the insomniacs and their healthy sleeper dopplegängers, the insomniacs actually had *more* deep sleep.

It boils down to this: The fact that the two groups had different biological responses (sometimes exactly opposite responses) even though they had matched sleep patterns, means that insomnia and sleep deprivation are not the same thing and do not have the same effect on people. It also means that whatever is causing the daytime symptoms of insomnia—greater feeling of tension, the tired-but-wired feeling—is not the lack of sleep, per se. It's something *else*. (Spoiler: it's hyperarousal, a concept we'll keep coming back to.)

(There are some exceptions where a person could have insomnia *and* be chronically sleep deprived. These cases include people who also have significant sleep apnea, other sleep disorders, and/or severe post-traumatic stress disorder, which can prevent them from getting enough sleep while also overriding sleepiness with hyperarousal. But even for these folks, insomnia can be treated.)

But how could you not be sleep-deprived when you, a person with insomnia, get so little sleep? Here are a few possible reasons:

1. **You may be getting too little sleep on some nights, but the average amount of sleep you get is close to adequate.**

- Other sleep disorders (e.g., obstructive sleep apnea)

- Other medical/psychiatric conditions that prevent sleep or increase hyper-arousal (e.g., PTSD, significant pain)

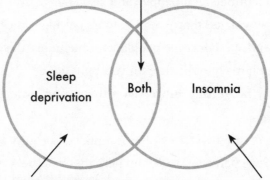

- Pulling all-nighters to study/party

- Not having enough time to sleep due to job/family obligations

- Significant disruptions from the environment (e.g., newborn who needs 24/7 care)

- Has enough opportunity to sleep

- No obvious external sleep disruptors

We tend to remember last night's sleep and the worst night's sleep, which is why most patients tell me they only sleep four hours per night, or five hours if they're lucky. However, once they start to keep a daily sleep log, they see that they sometimes sleep four to five hours and at other times they sleep six to seven hours, or maybe even more, if they start to count the times they go back to bed for half an hour after breakfast, or doze off in front of the TV for fifteen minutes after dinner. On occasion, they might even "crash" and get nine groggy hours after a run of three bad nights. This doesn't mean their sleep *quality* is great, nor that they feel rested, but the total amount of sleep they get over the course of a week or two may just be adequate enough that they're not sleep-deprived.

2. **You might not need as much sleep as you've been led to believe.**

    The previous chapter worked hard to bust the myth of eight hours as the required amount of sleep—in fact, sleep needs are different between people, and also change over time. You might be worried that your 6.5 hours per night means you're sleep-deprived. For some people, at some times, this would be true, but it may not be true for you right now.

3. **You may be getting more sleep than your brain is able to perceive.**

    One of the mysteries of insomnia is its ability to change the way we perceive sleep, and perhaps even the way we perceive time. We used to call it "paradoxical insomnia" when someone feels like they took hours to fall asleep, but measurements of their brain waves showed that it only took them twenty minutes. Now we know that this is a nearly universal experience for people with chronic insomnia, at least to some degree.

    No, I'm not saying that you're exaggerating your symptoms or that it's all in your head. Insomnia is as real as any other medical problem. I 100 percent believe your experience. I also know that the brain sometimes plays tricks with our perception, like when a stubbed toe can feel like the worst pain in the world for someone who just violently kicked their broken-down car, but can feel like no pain at all for the soccer player who just scored the winning World Cup goal.

    For people with insomnia, lighter stages of sleep (e.g., Stage 1 and Stage 2) can feel like no sleep at all, even as a sleep technologist watches the sleeper's brain waves do the exact same things that a healthy sleeper's brain does during the same sleep stages.* Remember how Stage 2 sleep is supposed to take up about half the night? That's a lot of opportunity to feel like you're not sleeping when your brain really is. Also, we don't perceive time passing when we're asleep because, well, we're unconscious. We may look at the clock and see 1:00 A.M., roll over feeling frustrated, try hard to fall asleep for a while, then look again after what seems like forever to see 2:00 A.M. Even though we may have been sleeping for *some* of the time in between, it feels like we've been awake for a full hour, especially because the passage of time itself feels slower when we're bored and frustrated.

REM sleep perception can also be affected. Usually, people feel like their sleep is deepest during REM, and lightest during non-REM.† But for people with the type of sleep perception common in insomnia, REM sleep does not feel deep and satisfying,‡ which robs them of a big chunk of the night (~25 percent) where they could be feeling like they're sleeping well.

Other factors tend to skew our overall estimation of how much sleep we get too. In a study of more than six thousand people,§ researchers found that asking someone to estimate

---

* A. G. Harvey and N. K. Tang, "(Mis) Perception of Sleep in Insomnia: A Puzzle and a Resolution," *Psychological Bulletin* 138, no. 1 (2012): 77.

† This is paradoxical because the reality of sleep depth is the opposite—REM is actually the lightest sleep and non-REM in the first few hours of the night is actually the deepest. This, again, goes to show how, even for healthy sleepers, perception versus reality can be complex.

‡ Aurélie M. Stephan, Sandro Lecci, Jacinthe Cataldi, and Francesca Siclari, "Conscious Experiences and High-Density EEG Patterns Predicting Subjective Sleep Depth," *Current Biology* 31, no. 24 (2021): 5487–5500. https://doi.org/10.1016/J.CUB.2021.10.012.

§ Christopher B. Miller, Christopher J. Gordon, Leanne Toubia, Delwyn J. Bartlett, Ronald R. Grunstein, Angela L. D'Rozario, and Nathaniel S. Marshall, "Agreement between Simple Questions about Sleep Duration and Sleep Diaries in a Large Online Survey," *Sleep Health* 1, no. 2 (2015): 133–37. https://doi.org/10.1016/J.SLEH.2015.02.007.

how much sleep they get in different ways can significantly change their answer. Specifically, if you ask someone, "On average, how many hours of sleep would you normally get," they would underestimate their nightly sleep duration by about twenty minutes compared to if you asked them to keep a sleep diary for seven days. This underestimation goes up to twenty-nine minutes if someone has depressive symptoms, thirty-five minutes if they have anxiety symptoms, and thirty-seven minutes if they have hypertension. Things like having other health conditions or not currently being employed can also exacerbate this effect. Unfortunately, people with insomnia tend to have more depression, anxiety, and other health concerns, so they're especially prone to feel like they get less sleep than they do.

But you're not doomed to this bizarre perceptual problem forever. Based on a huge analysis of thousands of insomnia patients' sleep before and after treatment, my colleagues and I have found that cognitive behavioral therapy for insomnia restores a much more accurate perception of sleep.

4. **It might be something other than "not enough sleep" that feels so bad.**

You may understandably protest, "But if you're right and I'm not really sleep-deprived, how come I feel the effects of sleep deprivation, like feeling tired, having trouble concentrating and remembering, having a short temper, and just feeling like I'm not functioning at 100 percent?"

Sleep deprivation could certainly cause those problems. But so can stress, fatigue, low mood, anxiety, desperation, boredom, worry . . . sound familiar? These are all ingredients in the insomnia soup.

Remember how insomnia is a twenty-four-hour disorder? It involves a hyped-up fight-or-flight system during both day and night, which is exhausting for your body. If you're frustrated that your sleep seems so unpredictable, anxious about it affecting your health, or sometimes even hopeless about ever getting good sleep again . . . all of this is exhausting too, not to mention distracting and irritating. No wonder you have trouble concentrating or don't feel like yourself. One of the best things about overcoming insomnia is that the weight of the anxiety, frustration, and hopelessness lifts, making it a lot easier to feel upbeat, sharp, and optimistic again.

Bonus: Sleep Hygiene Is Not the Answer to Insomnia

To understand what insomnia isn't, it's important to know what sleep hygiene isn't. In clinical trials for new drugs, researchers give some participants the real drug and some a sugar pill so they can see if the real drug performs better than the placebo. In clinical trials for insomnia, we give some participants the real treatment and some sleep hygiene instructions so we can see if the real treatment is better than the placebo. Yes, that's right. **Sleep hygiene is used as the placebo condition in many insomnia clinical trials because we know that it does not work for insomnia.**

You probably know the generic sleep hygiene rules pretty well, because I bet healthcare blogs have repeated them to you *ad nauseum*:

- Make your bedroom dark, quiet, and cool.
- Don't consume caffeine in the afternoon or evening.
- Don't exercise within several hours of bedtime.
- Don't eat a big meal close to bedtime.
- Don't use electronic devices/screens close to bedtime.
- Use your bed only for sleep and sex.
- Go to bed and wake up at the same time every day.
- Create a relaxing bedtime routine.

Now, if you do drink a Starbucks Venti coffee or two after dinner, or keep a loud TV show on all night in the bedroom . . . these are certainly habits to change (see chapter 11). If you do and your sleep problems go away, you'll know that you didn't have real insomnia in the first place, but rather an external chemical or environmental sleep disruptor. If you still have trouble falling or staying asleep when your sleep hygiene is generally good, you have bona fide insomnia, and sleep hygiene tips are not going to cure it.

Why doesn't sleep hygiene cure insomnia? It's for the same reason that dental hygiene (e.g., brushing your teeth, flossing) doesn't cure cavities. It's too little, too late. It's not that sleep hygiene tips are wrong. It's that most of them do not address the underlying problems of insomnia. For example, making the bedroom dark, quiet, and cool does generally improve conditions for sleep, but it's not going to help your insomnia much because your insomnia is almost certainly not due to your bedroom being too bright or noisy or hot. Some tips do address insomnia mechanisms, but when presented in this checklist format, without context or explanation, they don't end up being implemented the right way. For example, using the bed only for sleep/sex is one of the most important behavioral changes in insomnia therapy, but every single one of my insomnia patients who say they already follow this rule is doing it wrong. They're still using the bed for the worst possible non-sleep/non-sex activity—*trying really hard* to sleep. Chapters 5 and 9 will dive into why this and other common behaviors drive insomnia.

In fact, when implemented incorrectly, sleep hygiene rules may be even worse than useless, because some of them might actively backfire and make your insomnia worse. Whenever a patient comes into the clinic and leads with, "I have perfect sleep hygiene," I know that a big part of their insomnia is caused by Sleep Effort—the act of trying too hard and chasing sleep away as a result (chapter 9). For all of these reasons, following sleep hygiene rules is used as the placebo condition in insomnia clinical trials. This is why Hello Sleep is designed to fully unpack the sleep hygiene guidelines that will help you if you understand the rationale, reassure you about the ones that don't matter, and put the potentially dangerous ones into context so you don't sabotage your hard-won gains.

How Did I Develop Chronic Insomnia?

If everybody experiences a night of insomnia here or there, how come it only becomes a chronic problem for some people? If sleep hygiene is not the culprit nor the answer, what is? The story of the three Ps (predisposing factors, precipitating factors, and perpetuating factors)* will help you to understand.

Predisposing Factors

Some people are born a little more prone to insomnia than others, or experience things that make them more prone to insomnia very early in life. Perhaps they're a light sleeper who's sensitive to noise, or they tend to worry, or have a more trigger-happy fight-or-flight system. Perhaps they experienced trauma or never had the opportunity to learn healthy sleep patterns in childhood. Think of having these traits as having a stack of kindling—it gets you closer to having a fire, but it's not enough to actually make a flame.

Precipitating Factors

These are the things that come along and light the first spark for your insomnia. It could be a stressful job, a cross-country move, a new baby, win-

---

* A. J. Spielman, L. S. Caruso, and P. B. Glovinsky, "A Behavioral Perspective on Insomnia Treatment," *Psychiatric Clinics of North America* 10, no. 4 (1987): 541–53.

ning a big award, planning a wedding, going through a divorce, taking care of an elderly parent . . . there are infinite things that can trigger a bout of insomnia, and you may not even know what your precipitating factors were. But it doesn't really matter what set off the spark. Most of the time, either the stressor goes away, or we adjust to it, and sleep goes back to normal.

Perpetuating Factors

In the cases where insomnia continues or gets worse, taking on a life of its own beyond the original trigger, perpetuating factors are to blame. These are the logs we're continually adding onto the fire that keep the insomnia going, including the unhelpful things we do and the unhelpful ways we think about sleep.

You may protest that your sleep hygiene is great, so you don't have any unhelpful sleep habits acting as perpetuating factors. I assure you that sleep hygiene is not the main problem. Instead, perpetuating factors are often perfectly reasonable things we do to try to fix our sleep problems:

- Going to bed early after having a couple of particularly bad nights
- Prioritizing sleep in your life, and arranging activities and schedules accordingly
- Using meditation to try to fall back to sleep
- Avoiding stimulating things like exercise or the iPad in the evenings
- Using a sleep tracking device to evaluate your sleep
- Trying to find the ideal room temperature, bedtime routine, pillow, etc.

Do any of these sound familiar? It almost looks like the sleep hygiene checklist, right? **But as you'll come to learn, these seemingly**

helpful behaviors are often the fuel that keeps chronic insomnia going.

Luckily, perpetuating factors are the ones we can do something about. We can't change predisposing and precipitating factors—we'd need, at the least, a time machine for that. But perpetuating factors are simply things we do and think, which are squarely within our realm of influence. All we have to do is understand how they work, so we can take these logs out of the fire and allow insomnia to run out of fuel.

To get there, you'll likely have to make some adjustments that will be difficult at first. Know that these changes (or at least the discomfort that comes with them) are temporary. And they're very doable! It's not like losing weight and keeping it off, which will always require at least a little bit of vigilance and effort. Once you and sleep are friends again, your new ways of thinking and acting around sleep will not be effortful and should not require much attention at all.

In the next chapter we'll get all of your ducks in a row before plunging into part II, The Big Reset, where the real work will begin. To set you up for success, you'll do a quick self-assessment to see if you're ready for the Hello Sleep program. I'll also recommend a plan for handling sleep medications and gadgets before you start, and give you the most important tool from my tool belt—the sleep log.

BOTTOM LINE

- Chronic insomnia is a twenty-four-hour disorder. During the day, someone with insomnia is tired, stressed, tense, and/or moody. During the night, they have trouble falling or staying asleep.
- Insomnia is *not*
  » getting less than any specific amount of sleep;

» a chemical imbalance or malfunctioning brain area; or

» chronic sleep deprivation.

- Even though it may seem obvious that insomnia makes you sleep deprived, most people with insomnia are not, because

  » they might not need as much sleep as they've been led to believe;

  » they may be getting more sleep than their brain is able to perceive under the stress of insomnia;

  » they tend to remember their worst nights instead of average nights, so they may be getting more sleep overall than their initial impression; and

  » it might be something other than "not enough sleep" that feels so bad.

- Sleep hygiene is not the answer to insomnia—it is actually the placebo condition we use in insomnia clinical trials. It doesn't address the underlying problems, and may even backfire.

- Chronic insomnia progresses over time through the 3 Ps:

  » Predisposing factors—things that make you a little prone to insomnia, like being a light sleeper

  » Precipitating factors—things that trigger a bout of insomnia, like going through a divorce or losing a job

  » Perpetuating factors—things that keep insomnia going in the long run, which are often seemingly reasonable things we do to try to improve our sleep

- We can't control the first two Ps, but we *can* do something to undo the perpetuating factors. The next chapter will set you up for success before you dive into part II, which will begin to dismantle your perpetuating factors for insomnia.

3

Getting Ready for Your Hello Sleep Journey

Now that you know about sleep and insomnia in general, it's time to hone your own sleep and get ready for change.

Conditions don't have to be perfect for you to start sleep therapy. You don't have to wait for a totally stress-free month, defer traveling, or cancel major obligations. In fact, one important thing we're trying to achieve is not having to tiptoe around insomnia. Let's begin by acting exactly as we would if insomnia were not a part of life. How liberating that would be!

Of course, this is easier said than done. Insomnia has likely wedged itself into your daily decisions and routines in a few ways, and a couple of them should be addressed before you plunge into the Hello Sleep program:

- How you take (or don't take) sleep medications
- How you use sleep-related gadgets

What Should I Do About Sleep Medications?

You don't need to stop taking any medications to do this program. In fact, it's better to stay stable on your sleep medications and keep taking them as prescribed for now.* I know that for many of you, one major goal of insomnia therapy is to come off sleep drugs, and I want you to know that this is very doable. I have helped people taper off taking multiple nightly heavy-duty sleep drugs.

Chapter 10 will teach you how to do this (with the permission and support of the prescribing healthcare provider), in a way that minimizes withdrawal symptoms and maximizes the chances of long-term success. In general, please don't make any medication changes without consulting with your prescribing healthcare provider. In my experience, doctors are thrilled to hear that you want to stop taking sleep medications, but you always want to make sure that they approve of your plan before proceeding, because some medications are too dangerous to taper too quickly, or there might be other reasons your doctor wants you to stay on a certain medication.

Meanwhile, keep taking your medications as prescribed, **but do not use it as an emergency patch or play mental gymnastics with the dosage and frequency**. By this, I mean the nightly (or every-other-night or every-week) dance of, "Should I take it? But I already did last night. Should I take a half pill? Maybe try to wait until absolutely necessary? Oh, screw it, it's now 3:00 A.M. and I'm desperate." I know you're trying to take as little of your sleep medication as possible, but this angsty love-hate relationship with your drug is actually increasing your psychological dependence on it, likely prolonging its presence in your life.

---

* One possible exception is if your sleep feels perfect right now because you're taking a sleep aid nightly, and there's no room to improve without ditching the drug. In this case, you can choose to first taper off the medication using the method in chapter 10, but of course only with approval and guidance from your prescribing healthcare provider.

If you want to get off your sleep medication for good, you have to stop playing tug-of-war with it. **That means you should have a consistent sleep medication regimen**, whether it's full dose, nightly, at 9:00 P.M., or half dose on weekdays only at 10:00 P.M. or some other easy-to-follow routine. Be honest and generous with yourself—set a plan that you know you can stick to, without much temptation to add an extra "emergency" half pill at 3:00 a.m. Take your planned dose at the planned time even if you don't feel like you need it that night, and do *not* take anything you hadn't put in your plan, even if you feel like you really need it. No ifs, ands, or buts.

Commit to the plan for the duration of Hello Sleep, even if it feels like sleep is getting worse or better. And by the time you reach chapter 10, you will be ready to taper down. **This approach takes the uncertainty, guilt, hypervigilance, and love-hate angst out of the equation, which will ultimately help you overcome insomnia more easily.**

What Should I Do with Sleep Gadgets?

As a scientific researcher, I am very excited about consumer sleep trackers like Fitbit, Garmin, and Apple Watch. These devices give epidemiologists and sleep researchers access to huge amounts of real-life data, which allows us to understand sleep on a scale never before possible. But as a sleep therapist, especially one who works mostly with insomnia patients, I have mixed feelings about them. See if this sounds familiar:

Kate, the data engineer whose insomnia saps her energy and makes her feel like a zombie, is very good with numbers. Of course, she uses a sleep tracker. She wants to study the numbers and use them to crack the code. Every morning, the first thing she does is study her sleep report and compare it to her partner's. Sometimes she gets a glimmer of hope because her tracker tells her that she slept more than usual. Often, she feels frustrated and hopeless because she sees that she only got 9 percent deep sleep.

I have three main reservations about people with insomnia using consumer sleep trackers:

1. **The estimates may be inaccurate, likely in a way that could make your relationship with sleep worse.** The algorithms used to estimate sleep and sleep stages in these devices were based mostly on healthy sleepers' data. Until 2020, research studies had not been conducted showing how accurate these devices are in people with insomnia. It turns out that Fitbits, on average, underestimate deep sleep in people with insomnia (only catching it about half the time), and overestimate light sleep.*

2. **They don't tend to provide scientifically sound interpretations of the data, nor actionable advice based on the data.** Some devices give you an overall "sleep score," but this doesn't correspond to any medical standard or otherwise have any actionable meaning. Some devices give you estimates of time spent in each stage of sleep and how many times you woke up, but they don't say anything about what is considered healthy for each of these parameters or why, leaving you, again, without any concrete advice. You may feel terrible upon seeing what seems like a low percentage of deep sleep and twelve separate awakenings, not knowing that these numbers indicate perfectly normal sleep.

3. **The action of using a sleep tracker, in and of itself, may make your relationship with sleep worse.** Have you com-

* P. Kahawage, R. Jumabhoy, K. Hamill, M. de Zambotti, and S. P. Drummond, "Validity, Potential Clinical Utility, and Comparison of Consumer and Research-Grade Activity Trackers in Insomnia Disorder I: In-lab Validation Against Polysomnography," *Journal of Sleep Research* 29, no. 1 (2020): e12931.

pared your sleep score or stats with your bed partner's and felt bad? Or googled what happens if you don't get enough deep sleep, and gotten worried? Has getting a report about your sleep every day actually helped you to sleep better at night, or has it cemented your identity as a bad sleeper, instead? If so, you may be a victim of "orthosomnia,"* the condition of having insomnia due to, or exacerbated by, the act of tracking it. This behavior is a perpetuating factor for insomnia for many reasons, one being that it teaches you that somebody (or something) else knows your sleep better than you do, which is a huge barrier to having a good relationship with sleep.

This doesn't mean you can't ever use a sleep tracker for fun again. When you don't have chronic insomnia anymore, and your relationship with sleep is rock solid, you may get to a place where checking those numbers is just entertainment.† But for now, I strongly recommend you turn off the sleep tracking function or simply pause using your device.

Do I Have Any Conditions That Might Make the Hello Sleep Program Risky?

I strongly recommend working with a behavioral sleep medicine specialist who can tailor insomnia treatment if you have

- bipolar disorder, or high risk for bipolar disorder;
- a psychosis spectrum disorder (e.g., schizophrenia);
- a seizure disorder; or

---

* K. G. Baron, S. Abbott, N. Jao, N. Manalo, and R. Mullen, "Orthosomnia: Are Some Patients Taking the Quantified Self too Far?" *Journal of Clinical Sleep Medicine* 13, no. 2 (2017): 351–54.

† Because consumer sleep trackers are not FDA-approved for diagnosis or treatment, "entertainment" is exactly their purpose, according to companies that make them.

- a condition that makes you at high risk for falls (e.g., mobility problems, Parkinson's disease).

We're concerned about these disorders because sudden changes in sleep patterns can be risky for people who have them. For example, getting significantly less opportunity to sleep might trigger a manic episode for someone who is at risk for bipolar disorder. Getting up during the night can increase the risk of falling if someone has mobility limitations. Since we will be learning how to make changes to our sleep timing and behaviors in part II (The Big Reset), I'd feel a lot better if you ask your doctor whether you can proceed with specific sleep changes, or better yet, work one-on-one with a sleep specialist. What you learn in part III (Going Deeper into the Relationship) should be safe for all to practice.

Do I Have Another Sleep Disorder That Should Be Addressed First?

At this point, you should have a good idea of whether you have insomnia disorder. But there are many other sleep disorders out there; some can make insomnia worse, some can masquerade as insomnia, and some are higher priority problems that will require you to drop this book and call your doctor today. See if any of these apply to you:

1. **I am frequently very sleepy during the day.** The sleepiness is so severe that I'm falling asleep in inappropriate or dangerous situations, or it's interfering with my ability to fully participate in school or at work or in my social relationships.
2. **I have at least three or four of these: snoring loudly/frequently, gasping or stopping breathing during sleep, being overweight, being over fifty years old, being male, having high blood pressure, having a large collar size.** Bonus "or-

ange flags" include grinding teeth during sleep, regularly waking with headaches, and waking with dry mouth.

3. **I have bizarre nighttime experiences, such as sleepwalking, sleep terrors, sleep paralysis, hallucinations, acting out dreams, or violent behaviors while sleeping.** I've unintentionally hurt myself or others during these experiences, or they happen often enough to worry me.

4. **I have a strong urge to move my legs in the evenings.** It's not because I'm in a bad mood or I have a muscle cramp. I just feel discomfort or a "funny feeling" in my legs, and only moving them will relieve it.

5. **I have nightmares frequently**. It's so bad that I dread going to bed, or the nightmares have lingering, negative effects on my waking life.

6. **I am, by nature, a night owl.** If I didn't have morning obligations, I would go to bed much later and wake up much later than I currently do. Being able to live on this late-to-bed and late-to-rise schedule would solve my insomnia problems.

7. **I am a night- or rotating-shift worker, or I am often jetlagged due to frequent long-distance travel.**

If you agree with items 1 or 2, you may have obstructive sleep apnea, hypersomnia, or another sleep disorder that needs medical attention before attempting insomnia self-help.

Most people with insomnia are not extremely sleepy during the day. Excessive daytime sleepiness indicates something more than insomnia, such as sleep apnea, a hypersomnia disorder, or other medical problem. These should be your top priority, and you should only embark on the Hello Sleep program (parts II and III) when these conditions are ruled out or stabilized. Consult with your doctor as soon as possible.

If you agree with item 3, you may have parasomnia. You should consult with a sleep specialist while proceeding with this book with caution.

The material in this book should still be helpful to you if you have a parasomnia disorder *and* insomnia, but if working through part II of this book (The Big Reset) makes your bizarre sleep symptoms worse, stop limiting your time in bed and skip to part III. Meanwhile, consult your doctor about possible parasomnia symptoms.

If you agree with items 4–7, you may have some other sleep-related or circadian disruption in addition to insomnia. I recommend consulting with a sleep specialist while going ahead with the Hello Sleep program.

These items refer to restless legs syndrome, nightmare disorder, and circadian rhythm sleep-wake disorders (see chapter 16). You should know that if you have a severe case of one of these disorders, it can be hard to fully treat insomnia on your own. But you will likely still benefit from Hello Sleep, and there is no reason to avoid it. (By the way, these sleep disorders are treatable too!)

Ready to Dive In?

The next chapters will guide you through a transformation in the relationship between you and your sleep. Part II (The Big Reset), when done with full commitment, is your quickest path to reducing insomnia symptoms. Part III (Going Deeper into the Relationship) is important for taking you all the way to long-term, insomnia-free living and for preventing future chronic insomnia. The concepts and skills I'll teach you are based on a combination of:

Cognitive Behavioral Therapy for Insomnia

Cognitive behavioral therapy for insomnia (CBT-I) is the most scientifically researched insomnia intervention in existence. It is considered the first-line treatment by the AASM,* with at least seventy-five high-quality, randomized clinical trials supporting its efficacy. It works because it addresses the perpetuating factors for chronic insomnia—the behaviors and ways of thinking that keep us stuck in a bad relationship with sleep. It is not about "thinking positive" or "improving sleep hygiene." Instead, it is about becoming more accurate in your knowledge and perception of sleep, and changing your sleep behaviors in a way that resets your sleep physiology and biological clock.

Phototherapy, Chronotherapy, and Behavioral Activation

These three tools are evidence-based methods to align biological clocks, improve daytime functioning, and improve mood. I always incorporate these methods into my work with patients because insomnia is not just a nighttime sleep problem. It's a twenty-four-hour problem that needs daytime remedies too. Since we're here to approach sleep health holistically, these tools will be indispensable for rebuilding our relationships with sleep.

Elements of Mindfulness- and Acceptance-Based Practices

These skills are not just about using a meditation app to calm down. Instead, they are ways of relating to our bodies, thoughts, environments,

* Jack D. Edinger, J. Todd Arnedt, Suzanne M. Bertisch, Colleen E. Carney, John J. Harrington, Kenneth L. Lichstein, Michael J. Sateia, et al., "Behavioral and Psychological Treatments for Chronic Insomnia Disorder in Adults: An American Academy of Sleep Medicine Clinical Practice Guideline," *Journal of Clinical Sleep Medicine* 17, no. 2 (2021): 255–62. https://doi.org/10.5664/jcsm.8986.

and sleep that will fundamentally change you and your brain activity. Many of my patients believe they have already tried mindfulness without benefit to their sleep but realize through the Hello Sleep program that they were missing some crucial elements. Once enlightened, they have applied these skills to other areas of life, including relationship problems, stress, coping with chronic health issues, and general wellness.

My Own Toolbox, Built from Clinical Experience and Creative Tinkering

These are tidbits and strategies I wouldn't have been able to glean from academic research alone. My patients and I like them, and I hope you will too.

SOAPBOX MOMENT

Some exasperated new patients tell me that they've already tried CBT-I, and it didn't work despite months of hard work. The "months" part is already a clue that something was off. CBT-I should take about four to eight sessions when you work with an experienced behavioral sleep medicine specialist. These patients might not have responded to CBT-I because some complicating factor, such as untreated sleep apnea or PTSD, prevented bare-bones CBT-I from working well (see chapters 15 and 16 for what to do in these cases). There are also many well-intentioned healthcare providers who genuinely believe they are doing CBT-I with their patients, but are missing important insights. All of these skeptical "CBT-I graduates" that I've met ultimately benefited from a combination of full CBT-I and other Hello Sleep tools.

To get the most out of the Hello Sleep program, I recommend the following:

1. **Dedicate six to ten solid weeks to doing the Hello Sleep program.** Think of your self-guided insomnia journey as similar to completing a course of physical therapy, which involves doing progressive exercises that build on each other over the weeks. Rushing through the program in less than four weeks might not allow changes to really "sink in." Taking longer than twelve or so weeks might make you lose momentum, preventing you from benefiting as much as you could. Each chapter in parts II and III should take about one to two weeks to complete.

2. **Take time to fully work through each chapter in part II and part III.** Feel free to read ahead or bounce around chapters for your own curiosity, but for most people, working steadily and sequentially through these foundational chapters brings the most benefit. I recommend dedicating a regular couple of hours per week—say, Saturday mornings from 10 A.M. to noon—for "class" time, where you review homework, check your sleep data, tweak your time-in-bed window prescription, and perhaps read a new chapter. You'll accumulate a small checklist of weekly skills to practice.

3. **Use part IV as a supplemental reference.** These chapters delve into sleep changes over time, as well as specific medical/psychiatric conditions and life events that interact with sleep. They can be read any time, in any order, or skipped entirely if not relevant to you. But don't skip parts II and III. That would be like trying to build a house without a foundation.

4. **Don't get stuck on one chapter for more than a couple of weeks.** That chapter might simply not be that important for you, or you're not quite ready to implement it yet. Let its ideas percolate while you move on to the next foundational skill. You can always come back to a "stuck" chapter when you feel ready.

Don't Begin Hello Sleep Without Doing This First

You will begin your journey to healthy sleep with one crucial step: getting in the habit of completing daily sleep logs. The sleep log is a mini questionnaire you complete each morning about last night's sleep. It asks you things like, "When did you get into bed?" and "How long did it take you to fall asleep?"

I cannot emphasize this enough: you cannot do insomnia therapy, self-guided or otherwise, without *daily* sleep log data. The most foundational skills and concepts we talk about will be based on your sleep logs, because these skills will not work unless they're tailored to you. Doing sleep therapy without sleep logs would be like buying shoes online without knowing your size. Therefore, completing these every day is *the* most important thing you can do, starting today.

You have two options for how to complete the crucial sleep logs:

- **Traditional paper-and-pencil version (see the appendix for one that you can photocopy and use during the program).**
- **The free Consensus Sleep Diary app (see www.Consensus SleepDiary.com).** This is the much, *much* better option. It's easier to use, requires less time/effort, will have no calculation errors, and automatically plots your important data on a graph to show your progress over time. You don't even have to download anything, since the app runs in a regular internet browser that you can access from your computer, tablet, or smartphone.

CONSENSUS SLEEP DIARY, THE BEST THING SINCE SLICED BREAD

This is the *only* sleep log app I would recommend. It's designed by Dr. Colleen Carney, the brilliant sleep scholar who (together with her colleagues) united all behavioral sleep medicine with the publication of the Consensus Sleep Diary* in 2012. For the first time, we had a standard format for the sleep log, our most valuable tool in treating insomnia.

Now there's an app for it! It's free and easy to use, designed beautifully, and has no distracting frills. It doesn't give bad advice (you'd be surprised how many sleep apps do), and it displays your important sleep variables, already calculated and graphed for you, in a clear dashboard. Another great option is the smartphone app CBT-I Coach, which has a good sleep log function under the "My Sleep" tab. Using one of these digital sleep logs will save you a lot of time and headache.

Ideally, you'll want to complete each day's sleep log entry in the morning soon after waking, when your memory is fresh. **You'll need at least one week's worth of daily sleep log data to start calculating your time-in-bed window** (you'll see what this means and why it's important in chapter 4). And just as important, you should fill out sleep log entries based on your *estimates* of how long you were awake and how many times you woke up. **Please do *not* watch a clock or use your smartphone to note precise times**, because this will virtually guarantee sleeplessness. In fact, put your smartphone out of reach and throw a T-shirt over your alarm clock. You should not have any way to tell what time it is when you wake up during the night . . . and you don't need to, because once your morning alarm is set, you have zero need to know the time. How liberating is that? For your sleep logs, what we want is not precision or ultimate truth, but rather your own perception of your sleep. This perception is what will guide your necessary behavior change.

Are you ready? Get excited. Let's dive in next with the Big Reset.

---

* Colleen E. Carney, Daniel J. Buysse, Sonia Ancoli-Israel, Jack D. Edinger, Andrew D. Krystal, Kenneth L. Lichstein, and Charles M. Morin, "The Consensus Sleep Diary: Standardizing Prospective Sleep Self-Monitoring," *Sleep* 35, no. 2 (2012): 287–302. https://doi.org/10.5665/sleep.1642.

BOTTOM LINE

- To get the most out of insomnia therapy, you should consult a sleep physician to rule out other potential sleep disorders that could interfere. Excessive daytime sleepiness is a particularly big red flag, and assessing this should be top priority.

- If you are currently taking any medications to help you sleep, I highly recommend establishing a consistent and predetermined medication regimen (i.e., not making on-the-go decisions about whether, when, and how much to take). Make sure you consult with your prescribing healthcare provider before making changes with your medications.

- If you are currently using a sleep tracking device, I highly recommend pausing this until you no longer have chronic insomnia. The simple act of using one can actually make insomnia worse.

- Conditions don't have to be perfect for you to begin the Hello Sleep program. I do recommend committing to giving part II and part III of this book your steady attention for about eight weeks, with a couple of hours set aside per week for "class time," and at least a few minutes per day to complete homework. Usually, it goes best when you work through the program in sequence.

- The single most important thing you should begin doing right now is to complete daily sleep logs. You will complete one every day, at least for the first four weeks of the Hello Sleep program. The data from these sleep logs will serve as the foundation for a crucial part of insomnia therapy.

- Put your phone out of reach and cover up your alarm clock overnight. Stop clock-watching and simply use your best guesstimates to complete sleep logs.

PART II

The Big Reset

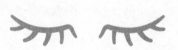

The Empty Piggy Bank

Why You Can't Fall (or Stay) Asleep

In any given moment, whether or not you will fall asleep boils down to the balance between two forces: sleep drive versus arousal. If you have more sleep drive than arousal right now, you will fall asleep soon. If you have more arousal than sleep drive, you won't.

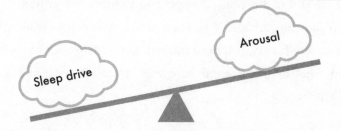

What Is Sleep Drive?

Homeostatic sleep drive* is your "hunger" for sleep. Just like the longer you go without eating, the more hunger (for food) builds up, the

---

* Alexander A. Borbély, Serge Daan, Anna Wirz-Justice, and Tom Deboer, "The Two-Process Model of Sleep Regulation: A Reappraisal," *Journal of Sleep Research* 25, no. 2 (2016): 131–43. https://doi.org/10.1111/JSR.12371.

longer you go without sleeping, the more homeostatic sleep drive builds up. If you just finished eating Thanksgiving dinner, you have zero hunger. If you just woke up from a full night of good quality sleep, you have zero sleep drive. At this point, your sleep drive piggy bank is empty.

Over the course of the day, you save up more and more sleep drive simply by being awake.* For every minute that passes where you're awake and doing stuff, you're putting a coin in your piggy bank of sleep drive. You're putting away bonus coins if you're physically active. At bedtime, hopefully you have saved up enough in your piggy bank to buy a good night's sleep.

What happens when you don't have enough sleep drive saved up? For most adults, it takes about sixteen to eighteen hours of being awake to save enough in the piggy bank for a good quality sleep.† You've probably spent time wondering how many hours of sleep you need to function well during the day. But you may never have wondered how many hours of daytime functioning you need to earn good sleep. Of course, this fluctuates over time and depends on your developmental stage and current lifestyle. If you're a teenage competitive swimmer, you need less time to fill up your piggy bank. If you're a retiree who enjoys reading history books in a dim library, you need more time to fill up your piggy bank.

Now, what might be some sure ways to sabotage your sleep drive piggy bank?

---

* On an oversimplified biological level, the homeostatic sleep drive reflects the accumulation of adenosine in the brain. Adenosine is a neurochemical, and it's essentially a by-product of energy consumption. Sometimes patients ask if they can take an adenosine pill to get more sleep drive. Sadly, this is not possible. Sleep drive is not bought, but earned.

† It would take less than this if you're LeBron James because he engages in extremely high levels of physical exertion, which may translate to needing only, say, twelve hours to save enough sleep drive in his piggy bank.

Sabotage #1: Going to Bed Too Early

One of the most common things my insomnia patients do is go to bed too early. This is very understandable, of course, because they want to make up for last night's poor sleep; or because "10:30 P.M. seems like a decent hour to go to bed"; or because "this is when I've always gone to bed." If your bedtime is based on something arbitrary, like your partner's bedtime or on a lack of better options or even your personal historical precedent, you may not have saved up enough sleep drive in your piggy bank.

Often, my patients very earnestly feel that they must have enough sleep drive saved up, because they feel *so* tired they don't see any option other than going to bed. **But there is a crucial difference between tired and sleepy.**

Feeling *tired* means feeling worn out, depleted, exhausted, bored, low energy, "done with the day" . . . it's your body and mind asking for rest, rejuvenation, or sometimes, just a change of scenery. In moments like these, the cure may be a nice stretch, a comforting cup of tea, or a walk in the park.

Feeling *sleepy* means you're close to falling asleep. That's it. If your eyes are drooping and your head is involuntarily nodding, or you've been missing plot points in the movie you're watching . . . you are sleepy. In this case, the cure is to sleep.

You may very well be tired but not sleepy, and if that's when you go to bed, you probably don't have enough sleep drive in your piggy bank yet to pay for a good night's sleep. Instead, you'd be buying yourself lots of tossing and turning, being easily woken up, and feeling frustrated. Of course, that doesn't mean we should just ignore fatigue— it's always important to listen to your body and respond to its needs. It's just that trying to sleep is not a particularly good cure for fatigue. It may even backfire by preventing you from saving up more sleep drive in the piggy bank, leading to more difficulty falling or staying asleep.

Sabotage #2: Lingering in Bed in the Morning

Some of my patients love to linger in bed in the morning, which I can very much relate to. There is nothing cozier than hanging out in bed before the hubbub of the day starts. For some, it's not even about the luxury of lying in. Perhaps their piggy bank ran empty long before their alarm clock went off in the morning, and they linger in bed hoping to catch just a little more sleep. They end up scraping together enough sleep drive to doze on and off for an extra hour, skimming the surface of sleep. But this is borrowing against today's piggy bank balance and starting their savings too late in the day. **They still end up feeling unsatisfied with their sleep quality, and now they also find themselves in a cycle of perpetually low sleep drive balance.**

Sabotage #3: Alternating Between Short and Long Nights

Another pattern I see is the feast-or-famine sleep drive balance. Someone spends two or three nights struggling a lot and sleeping very little, then they crash and "make up" for it by spending ten hours in bed for a night or two, catching eight or nine groggy hours. Sometimes this makes them feel amazing and they believe this means eight to nine hours is what they need every night.* Sometimes they wake up feeling even worse. Either way, now they've really gone into the red with their sleep drive balance, because not only did they overspend last night, they've

---

* This is like enjoying three steaks and a loaf of bread after a week-long hunger strike and believing this means three steaks and a loaf of bread is what you need for every meal.

also got less time today to save up sleep drive for tonight's sleep, so they pay for it with another run of tough nights, then another crash . . . and the cycle begins again.

Sometimes when we look at a patient's sleep log over the course of a week or two, we see that on average, they're getting a pretty decent amount of sleep—perhaps more than they would have guessed. And yet they say, "If only I could get six and a half solid hours of sleep *every* night, instead of swinging between four-and-a-half-hour nights and eight-and-a-half-hour nights . . . I'd be alright."

They're right! Having a consistent sleep-wake pattern and consistently good quality sleep *is* much healthier than going through feast-or-famine with your sleep, even if the average amount of sleep over a week is the same. But if you keep making up for bad nights by over-spending time in bed, you won't be able to get off your wildly swinging pendulum.

Sabotage #4: Being Inactive During the Day

See if this sounds familiar: You wake up after a bad night feeling not at all rested. If anything, you feel more tired and frazzled than when you went to bed last night. You feel so lousy and low-energy that you throw in the towel on the day. Either you cancel plans in order to recover, or lay around as much as possible to "save up energy" for the things you have to do. You can't muster up the energy to run nonessential errands or try to get together with friends.

As bedtime approaches, you think to yourself, "Surely I'm exhausted enough, after such a brutal night last night, that I'll sleep well tonight," only to find that when your head hits the pillow, your body has some-how found a second wind. You toss and turn and feel so tired and yet so wired.

So, what's happened here? Well, there's not enough information to tell why that first night was so awful. But the next day, we can see how lying on the couch and forfeiting physical/social activity could sabotage that day's sleep drive savings. This kind of day is not only one of low physical exertion, which doesn't earn you a lot of sleep drive, it's also one of low mental and social stimulation, which can feed boredom, a "blah" mood, and ironically, fatigue. What we end up with is a double-whammy of not saving up enough sleep drive *and* feeling even more physically and emotionally lousy. Does this sound like a combination that leads to a satisfying fall into blissful sleep?

Now extend this scenario from day to day, week to week, year to year. You're not being a couch potato every day, probably. But how many days do you feel like you've truly lived to the fullest—physically, mentally, and socially—in the past year? How many have you wasted by lying on the couch with Netflix instead of getting active? It's not that you have to be busy all the time . . as you'll learn later in the book, daytime rest is necessary for healthy sleep. But even good quality rest, such as taking a walk or doing a hobby, involves engaging your body and mind.

I'm here to let you in on the counterintuitive secret that lousy, tired days are not the chicken. At this point, they're the egg. They may feel like the consequence of insomnia, but in fact, they are more the cause.

And don't worry, you don't need to take up triathlon training to earn that sleep drive during the day. Many of us nonathletes save enough in our piggy banks just fine. But if you're usually a couch potato, it may surprise you how much a daily walk around the neighborhood or a weekly lunch date with friends will do. And when you catch yourself using insomnia as an excuse to not do something, it's a good sign that you should *especially* go and do that thing.

SELF-REFLECTION

Do you save up enough sleep drive in your piggy bank during the day? If you're not sure, take a look at your sleep logs so far and ask yourself these questions:

- Am I sleepy (not just tired, but *sleepy*) by the time I go to bed?
- How do I decide when it's time for bed? Is it because I feel sleepy, or because of some other reason (e.g., it's my habit, because my partner does, because I think I should)?
- How long do I spend in bed each night? Is this very different between weekdays and weekends?
- How long do I spend out of bed each day? How do I spend that time?

Take your time to consider these questions. Make sure you consult your sleep log and use a calculator if you've completed the paper-and-pencil version, because often our general impression about when we go to bed or get up in the morning don't capture the whole picture. You'd be surprised at how many people are adamant that they "wake up, on the dot, at 6:57 A.M. every single day," but are simply remembering this interesting coincidence because it happened three days in a row last week . . . and the other four days they woke up after 7:30 A.M. and didn't get out of bed until after 7:45 a.m. The same goes for bedtimes—we're surprisingly bad at remembering nights other than last night and the worst night.

What Does This All Mean for My Sleep?

We can begin to compile our list of perpetuating factors for chronic insomnia now that we know about the sleep drive piggy bank and the things that can sabotage it:

- Going to bed too early
- Spending too long in bed
- Trying to make up for bad nights by "crashing" every few nights
- Being too inactive during the day

If any of these are true for you, then no wonder you're not getting better sleep. Expecting yourself to sleep well without enough sleep drive is like only putting half a tank of gas in the car and expecting to drive a full tank's distance. Although we each have different overall sleep needs depending on our age, lifestyle, and other factors, what we all have in common is that our day-to-day behaviors affect how much we have in our own unique sleep drive piggy bank each day. It doesn't matter if you're a twenty-year-old varsity athlete or ninety-year-old nursing home resident—these perpetuating factors will sabotage your sleep drive and make it hard for you to have a good relationship with your sleep.

Don't be mad at your sleep for not taking you as far as you'd like. After all, your car can only run on the fuel it's given, and your sleep can only run on the sleep drive it's given. Instead of blaming sleep for not performing for you, let's see what we can do to help by asking, "Hello Sleep, my friend. How can I help increase the sleep drive you need?"

How to Increase Sleep Drive (Sleep Consolidation)

You may have guessed that the best way to increase your sleep drive is to spend less time in bed, which we can call sleep consolidation.* This accomplishes two things:

---

* A. J. Spielman, P. Saskin, and M. J. Thorpy, "Treatment of Chronic Insomnia by Restriction of Time in Bed," *Sleep* 10, no. 1 (1987): 45–56.

1. You have more time being out of bed to save up sleep drive.
2. You have less time to overspend your sleep drive while lying in bed.

If we also add spending more consistent amounts of time in bed from night to night, at more consistent times, we accomplish even more:

3. You develop a predictable rhythm that your biological clock will love. The better your clock can predict the timing of day versus night, the better it can help you to sleep and wake.

We've known for decades that sleep consolidation is the surest way to decrease insomnia. Recent research* confirms that a four-week sleep consolidation treatment works exactly how we think it does—by increasing sleep drive and decreasing arousal. That's why we start the Big Reset with sleep consolidation—it's our most efficient tool for tipping the scales in sleep's favor.

What's the Right Amount of Time to Spend in Bed?

There isn't one "right" amount of time to spend in bed for everyone, because all of us have different sleep needs. Over time, you'll learn to listen to your body's needs and know your personal answer intuitively. For now, only your sleep logs will be able to give you a specific number. By now, you hopefully have at least one full week (ideally, two) of sleep logs. They should have chronicled when you went to bed each

---

* Leonie F. Maurer, Colin A. Espie, Ximena Omlin, Richard Emsley, and Simon D. Kyle, "The Effect of Sleep Restriction Therapy for Insomnia on Sleep Pressure and Arousal: A Randomised Controlled Mechanistic Trial," *Sleep* 45, no. 1 (January 2022): zsab223. https://doi.org/10.1093/SLEEP/ZSAB223.

night, how long it took you to fall asleep, how many times you woke up, etc. Using these logs, you can calculate a few important variables that we will keep coming back to in the coming weeks. It's worth spending some time to understand them now.

Step 1: Understand Your Sleep Log Numbers
(See the Appendix for Examples)

Time in Bed

This is how much time you physically spent in bed last night. More accurate, it's the total block of time from the moment you physically got into bed to the moment you physically got out of bed to start your day the next morning. Let's say you physically got into bed at 11:00 P.M. last night and immediately turned the lights out to try to sleep, took a while to fall asleep, got up to use the bathroom in the night, woke up at 5:30 A.M. to your cat screaming at you, fed her quickly but got back into bed to try to get back to sleep (unsuccessfully) for a while, eventually giving up and getting out of bed to shower at 7:00 A.M. Your total time in bed last night was eight hours (from 11:00 P.M. to 7:00 A.M.). Never mind about the five minutes you got out of bed to feed the cat—that was still within the block of time when you were trying to sleep, similar to a bathroom break during the night.

Time to Fall Asleep

This refers to how long it took you to fall asleep once you started trying (sitting in bed watching TV or doing another activity doesn't count). If you physically got into bed at 11:00 P.M., read for fifteen minutes before turning out the lights to try to sleep at 11:15 P.M., and fell asleep at about 11:45 P.M. . . . . your time to fall asleep was thirty minutes (from 11:15 P.M. to11:45 P.M.).

Time Awake During the Night

This is the total amount of time you spent awake during the night after you initially fell asleep. If you turned the lights out at 11:15 P.M., took thirty minutes to fall asleep, and eventually got woken by your alarm at 7:00 A.M., you'd count all the time you spent awake between falling asleep at 11:45 P.M. and waking up at 7:00 a.m. Perhaps you got up and used the bathroom for five minutes in the middle of the night, and woke again at some point and couldn't get back to sleep for ninety minutes. Add those up (5 minutes + 90 minutes = 95 minutes), and you've got a total "time awake during the night" of ninety-five minutes.

Total Sleep Time

This is how much sleep you actually got. If we start with your total sleep opportunity (from lights out to your final awakening), then take away time to fall asleep, and take away time awake during the night, we should be left with your total sleep time. Lights out was at 11:15 P.M. and your alarm woke you up at 7:00 a.m . . . that's seven hours and forty-five minutes total opportunity to sleep. Take away thirty minutes of time to fall asleep, and take away ninety-five minutes of time awake during the night, and we're left with five hours and forty minutes of total sleep time (7 hours 45 minutes – 30 minutes – 95 minutes = 5 hours and 40 minutes).

Sleep Efficiency

This is the most interesting variable. Sleep efficiency refers to the percentage of time you're asleep during your time-in-bed block. In other words, out of the whole stretch of the night that you spent in bed, what percentage of that time were you actually sleeping? In our example, you spent eight hours in bed (from 11:00 P.M. to 7:00 A.M.) but only had five hours and forty minutes total sleep time. Your sleep efficiency would be 71 percent (5 hours and 40 minutes ÷ 8 hours × 100 percent = 71 percent).

For once, I do have a specific number (or range) to offer: **A healthy average sleep efficiency is usually between 85 percent and 95 percent.** This means that the vast majority of the time you're in bed, you're sleeping. But it shouldn't be 100 percent because that would mean you conked out immediately upon getting horizontal, and was out like a dead log all the way until something yanked you out of bed the next day. If this happens more than occasionally, you should be concerned. It would mean you are not getting enough opportunity to sleep, or a different sleep disorder (one that is not insomnia) is causing you to be excessively sleepy.

If someone's sleep efficiency is pretty consistently in the 85 percent to 95 percent zone, they likely don't have insomnia. If it's often below 85 percent, or they average lower than 85 percent across a couple of weeks, they almost certainly have insomnia. One of our main tasks for the next few chapters is to keep an eye on your weekly average sleep efficiency—this will be our guide for how to tailor the Big Reset to you.

USE THE CONSENSUS SLEEP DIARY!

If you're still using a paper-and-pencil version of the sleep log, or another sleep diary/log app, I highly recommend that you switch to either the free Consensus Sleep Diary at www.ConsensusSleepDiary.com or the CBT-I Coach app. Other apps may very well lead you astray with poorly phrased questions, erroneous ways of calculating variables, plain wrong advice, or terrible designs that unnecessarily increase your anxiety about sleep. These things are not trivial.

If you're still relying on a wearable sleep tracker (e.g., Fitbit*) to

---

* Even if a wearable sleep tracker were accurate, which it often isn't, especially for people with insomnia, they do not reflect your own perception of your sleep duration/quality, and your perception is what we need to work with here. By the way, I have no affiliations with Fitbit or any company that makes sleep trackers.

produce your sleep variables, I am sad, because you are not getting what you should be out of this book. Everything here hinges on your *own* experience of your sleep, not what a movement detector inferred about your sleep. Stop using that wearable tracker today until you don't have chronic insomnia anymore.

Step 2: Calculate Your New Time-in-Bed Window

If you're using the Consensus Sleep Diary app, you already know your important sleep variables (see the "Sleep Data" tab). If you must use the paper-and-pencil sleep log, please see the appendix in this book for how to calculate time in bed, total sleep time, and sleep efficiency—these are the sleep variables you'll need.

Now, the fun part: we're going to make some Chicago-style deep dish pizza (a.k.a., we're going to consolidate your sleep). Here's what I mean: If you're making pizza from scratch, you have to make a crust out of dough. If you try to make the pizza too big, there won't be enough dough to go around, and you'll end up with a thin crust full of holes. Not a good pizza, and not the shape we want for our sleep, either. Instead, let's make a smaller pizza (i.e., smaller time-in-bed window), so we can have enough dough for a thick, even crust (i.e., enough sleep drive for a good quality night of sleep).

Here's how:

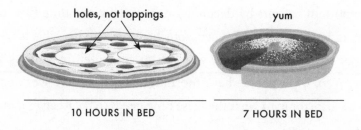

holes, not toppings · yum

10 HOURS IN BED · 7 HOURS IN BED

1. Note your average total sleep time in the past week. Let's say six hours and fifteen minutes.

2. Add thirty minutes to this average total sleep time. In this case, 6 hours and 15 minutes + 30 minutes = 6 hours and 45 minutes.

3. This is your new time-in-bed window, that is, the amount of time you're allowed to physically spend in bed per night. In this case, you're allowed to spend six hours and forty-five minutes in bed.

4. Note: Don't make this time-in-bed window less than five hours. For example, if your average total sleep time is four hours, just set your time-in-bed window to five hours.

IMPORTANT

If you do not have at least one week of sleep logs to work with, *do not guesstimate your average time in bed or total sleep time on your own.* People with insomnia, including very intelligent and rational people with great memories, tend to remember most vividly their worst nights and their most recent nights, which skews the average. We can't afford to be wrong about this average right now because it directly determines your sleep schedule for the next week or two at least. Spoiler: if you underestimate your average total sleep time too much, you're really going to hate next week.

Step 3: Decide When This Time-in-Bed Window Will Fall

It's important to start by deciding on your daily rise time first, before counting backward to see when your bedtime will be. This is because you can better control when you get up compared to when you fall asleep. Also, most people have morning obligations like work or kids, which will factor in to what their rise time needs to be. Keep in mind that you will need to get up at this time every day for at least the next couple of weeks, including days off work. Here's what I recommend:

- If possible, go with your natural wake time. If you usually wake without an alarm at 7:30 A.M., stick with that.
- If you must be up before your naturally preferred wake time (e.g., to take the kids to school), choose the latest time you can get up. Streamline your morning routine so you can give yourself more time to sleep.
- Don't choose an arbitrarily early rise time just because you believe early risers are better people or you have grand plans for becoming "more productive." There is nothing inherently better or more productive about getting up early. You'll do your personal best if you work with, instead of against, your body's natural preference.
- Don't choose a rise time so late that you're surely going to naturally wake up before then. For example, if you almost always naturally wake before 7:00 A.M., do not choose a rise time for 8:00 A.M.
- If you currently have no consistent wake time, or have no idea what your body's natural wake time would be if it had the choice, choose a rise time that seems most feasible.

Once you've chosen your daily rise time, do the following:

- **Set a daily morning alarm for this rise time.** Even if you're not in the habit of using an alarm clock, use one now. You'd be surprised at how many people undergoing the Big Reset start oversleeping their intended rise time, or keep waking up worried that they'll oversleep.
- **Calculate your earliest allowed bedtime.** For example, if your time-in-bed window is six hours and forty-five minutes, and your

chosen rise time is 6:45 A.M., then your earliest allowed bedtime is 12:00 midnight. If your chosen rise time is 6:00 A.M., then your earliest allowed bedtime is 11:15 P.M.

In Summary, Here Are Your Tasks for This Week:

1. Get up at your regular rise time every day: _____.
2. Don't go to bed until your earliest allowed bedtime: _____, or until you're sleepy, whichever is *later*.
3. Don't nap or "make up" for a bad night by sleeping in or going to bed early. In other words, no matter how your sleep goes, you must be up by your rise time, and you are not allowed in bed again until your earliest allowed bedtime.

What Exactly Do "Bedtime" and "Rise Time" Mean?

Bedtime refers to the time you physically get into bed in the evening, and rise time refers to the time you physically get out of bed. Let yourself linger for five minutes in the morning, if needed, to get your bearings and fire up the body's engines, but "rise" really does mean starting the day out of bed!

So, I Can't Sleep in at All on Weekends?

If it will help you to generally stick to the Big Reset protocol, we can allow for one hour of wiggle room on your days off. If your regular rise time is 6:00 A.M., then you can set your alarm to 7:00 A.M. on days off, but no later than that. This doesn't mean you have to stay in bed until your alarm, whether it's set to 6:00 A.M. or 7:00 A.M. If you naturally wake thirty minutes before your weekend 7:00 A.M. alarm, you should get up right away, with the happy knowledge that you will have a thirty-minute head start to saving up sleep drive for the day.

Won't I Become Even More Sleep-Deprived than I Already Am?

In chapter 2, we busted the myth of insomnia being the same thing as sleep deprivation. Very brief reminder: if you have insomnia, it's unlikely that you're sleep-deprived in general, because if you were sleep-deprived, you'd be too sleepy to have insomnia! Be reassured that you're unlikely to be starting from a place of sleep deprivation. But during the Big Reset phase, you may indeed become (temporarily and mildly) sleep-deprived, since your brain may not immediately learn to fill 85 to 95 percent of your time-in-bed window with good quality sleep. But this is okay. In fact, it's the whole point. We're trying to jump-start your sleep drive system, teaching your brain and body what it feels like to be sleepy again. Don't worry, you don't need to keep up this schedule forever.

What If I'm Really, Really Tired Before My Earliest Allowable Bedtime?

First, quick refresher: *tired* and *sleepy* are two completely different things. Tired means you've had a long day, you're bored, you've been stressed, you need a break, etc. Sleepy means you're about to fall asleep. Often, when evening rolls around and we long to crawl into bed, what we're longing for is closure to the day, escape from the big bad world, or simply a well-deserved rest. I feel this way as early as 7:30 P.M., when my toddler is finally in bed! That doesn't mean I'm *sleepy* at this time. Please do feel free to rest and indulge in whatever activity makes you feel relaxed and cozy in the evening, but don't go to bed unless you're truly *sleepy*.

If you're truly *sleepy* well before your earliest allowable bedtime . . . good! That means it's working. The Big Reset phase is all about making you sleepier than you need to be by bedtime. Remember, you're not following this schedule forever. Once you're better at telling true sleepiness from "false alarms," and your brain relearns how to do quality nighttime sleep . . . you *should* listen to your body's needs and go to bed when you're sleepy. For now, soldier on and wait until your earliest allowable bedtime.

But If I Miss My Sleepy Window at 9:00 P.M., I Will Get a Second Wind and Never Fall Asleep.

I often hear about this phenomenon from people with and without insomnia. But "missing my sleepy window" is actually a misunderstanding of what's happening. Feeling sleepy at 9:00 P.M. doesn't mean your body is actually ready for a full night's sleep. It's simply a vestige of our evolutionary past when our ancestors used to go to sleep not long after sunset. But they also used to get up at dawn, and as recently as preindustrial times in Europe, they used to spend a couple of hours awake in the middle of the night, doing chores and socializing. If you'd like to live this lifestyle, and you consistently stick with dawn as rise time, 1:00 A.M. as the cooking hour, and hard physical labor throughout the day, then you can happily go to bed at 8:00 P.M. with enough sleep drive saved for a rich night's sleep.

But if you live like most modern humans in the industrialized world, your 9:00 P.M. "sleepy window" is a false alarm. If you go to bed during this window, it's no wonder that you either have trouble falling asleep, or wake up at 2:00 A.M., having run out of sleep drive. And if that doesn't happen tonight, it probably will tomorrow night. Your subsequent "second wind" at 10:00 P.M. is simply your body getting past this false alarm, realizing that you're not really ready for bed yet.

Really, No Naps at All?

I love naps. Napping is my love language. In the long run, when you no longer have chronic insomnia, I will fully encourage you to take naps (or even adopt a full siesta habit!). But for now, we want to temporarily avoid naps in order to supercharge the effect of Sleep Consolidation. Right now, taking naps would be like stealing a little bit every day from your own piggy bank, so it's better to work through the urge and look forward to being sleepier at bedtime.

However, if you need to take a nap for safety, such as when you are feeling drowsy while driving, please do take a short nap. If you feel so sleepy after lunch that your eyes can't stay open, and it's going to ruin your day if you don't relieve yourself of this crushing sleepiness, go ahead and take a short nap even if you're not driving (also see chapter 15 for modifications to the no-napping rule for people with other psychiatric and medical conditions). Just set yourself a timer for thirty minutes so you can get a refresher but not steal too much from the piggy bank. If you're frequently this sleepy during the day, insomnia is not your main sleep problem, and you should talk to your doctor about other possible sleep disorders (see chapter 16).

If you're thinking, "A thirty-minute timer for a nap? But if I won't even fall asleep within thirty minutes," or, "By the time the timer goes off, I'll have *just* fallen asleep," then you're not sleepy enough to be taking a nap. You should only be breaking this emergency glass if you're irresistibly sleepy *right now*, to the point of it being a safety risk.

If I Have a Particularly Bad Night, or an Important Day Ahead, Can I Please Sleep in Late or Go to Bed Early?

The short answer is "no." Remember that feast-or-famine pattern that keeps you stuck in a vicious insomnia cycle? If you want to avoid famine, the only way to do it is to not feast. Get up at your regular rise time, and stay up until your bedtime, with the assurance that you'll be extra rich tonight (or tomorrow night) with sleep drive. And this abundance of sleep drive will pay off in the form of better quality sleep in the nights ahead. Sticking to your schedule during the Big Reset phase also regularizes your circadian rhythm (more on this in chapter 6), an important force for sleep health that many people overlook.

One possible caveat: if you're so sleepy during the day that you're nodding off in inappropriate situations or fighting tooth and nail to stay awake while driving, and this is unusual for you, take a short nap in the afternoon or go to bed slightly earlier (approximately by thirty minutes). If you're frequently this sleepy during the day, you should talk to your doctor about sleep disorders other than insomnia.

Can I Read or Do Other Stuff in Bed?

For now, you can do whatever you want in bed, as long as you don't spend more than your allowed time physically in bed. If you'd like to allocate some of your time-in-bed window to reading in bed, watching the news in bed, or playing an iPad game . . . go for it! But whatever you do or don't do in bed, you're not allowed to physically get into it until your bedtime, and you have to be physically out of it by rise time.

Should I Adjust My Time-in-Bed Window as the Week Goes On?

Stick to your time-in-bed window for at least a week. In the next chapter, you will learn to use your new sleep log data to tweak your window. You'll need at least one week's worth of data, so it's crucial to continue doing your sleep logs every day.

This All Sounds Miserable. Do I Need to Do This Forever?

Absolutely not. This is not meant to be a rest-of-your-life approach to sleep. In fact, the whole point of this book is to get you to a point, hopefully within a few weeks, where you don't have to run your sleep routine like a drill sergeant. We're only doing the Big Reset now because insomnia has taken you so far from your natural relationship with sleep that we wouldn't know where else to begin. This is a temporary measure to show your body what it feels like to be sleepy—a feeling that hasn't been coming naturally—and to teach your brain to fill sleep opportunity with quality sleep, instead of dilly-dallying all night with patchy, poor quality sleep. Once your sleep *quality* improves, *quantity* will follow.

The ultimate goal is to live in harmony with your sleep, in a way where you don't have to follow strict rules or do mental calculations about it. This type of relationship is much, much easier to achieve once we've hit the Big Reset button.

Does Caffeine Affect My Sleep Drive?

Yes, temporarily. See chapter 11 for a deep dive on how caffeine works and what this means for you. In short: Caffeine molecules take up the same docking sites on brain cells that adenosine, the sleep drive chemical, docks. Therefore, having too much caffeine prevents adenosine from docking and letting your brain know how much sleep drive is accumulating, which tricks your brain into not feeling sleepy when you truly are. That's why we generally don't want to drink coffee in the evenings or have too much overall. It's hard to say specifically how much you can have because there's a huge range in how sensitive people are to caffeine and how long it lasts in their system. If you're curious, you can always cut down on coffee or switch to decaf (gradually, so you're not hit with terrible withdrawal symptoms).

What About My Racing Mind?

Excellent question. The next several chapters are all about hyperarousal, much of which involves the racing-mind phenomenon so common in insomnia. For now, know that you'll already be decreasing the amount of time you spend with your racing mind simply by increasing your sleep drive.

BOTTOM LINE

- Your need and ability to sleep is based on the balance between your sleep drive and arousal. This chapter focused on sleep drive, which accumulates in your sleep drive piggy bank when you are awake and is spent when you sleep.
- Your sleep drive piggy bank can have a low balance for a few reasons:
  » You go to bed too early, before you've had enough time to save up enough sleep drive.
  » You linger in bed in the morning, which decreases the amount of time you have to save sleep drive during the day.
  » You take naps during the day, which is like stealing from your own piggy bank.
  » Your sleep has a feast-or-famine pattern, which keeps you in a cycle of overspending versus underspending your sleep drive.
  » You're not active enough during the day to earn enough sleep drive.
- To increase your sleep drive, spend less time in bed and follow your Big Reset schedule.
- To calculate your Big Reset schedule, use your daily sleep log data (you should have at least one week's worth of sleep logs to do this step):
  » Add thirty minutes to your average total sleep time, and this is your allowable time-in-bed window.
  » Decide when you want to get up each day (and every day).

- » Count backward from this rise time to see when you're allowed to get into bed.
- » Note: You don't *have to* get into bed at your calculated bedtime. You're just not allowed in bed before then.
- The more closely you follow your new schedule, with consistent rise times each morning and only spending your allowed time-in-bed window in bed, the more quickly your brain will begin filling your night with good quality sleep. Once the quality improves, quantity will follow.
- The next chapter will be all about the other side of the balancing equation—arousal.

The Drooling Dog

Why Your Brain Turns "On" at Night

In the last chapter, we introduced sleep drive, the sleepiness you deposit into your sleep drive piggy bank during the day and use to buy quality sleep at night. You need to be awake and out of bed long enough to save sufficiently for your sleep drive account. But sometimes, you work your butt off all day in the garden, or stay up later than usual, ending up exhausted by bedtime, but somehow still have trouble falling or staying asleep. What's going on?

Sleep drive is only half of the equation. It's the more straightforward half and the easier one to address, which is why we started our Big Reset there. And now it's time to take a look at the other side: arousal.

Arousal is simply being revved up—physically, mentally, or emotionally. It works against sleep drive. This is a good thing. Even if you spent all day hunting and gathering, earning yourself plenty of sleepiness, you'd still want an emergency override at bedtime if you saw a tiger stalking closer, right? In that moment, arousal from fear revs up your body and mind, making you ready to fight or flee. In this instance, arousal is a life-saving friend. **But too much of a good thing—especially at the wrong**

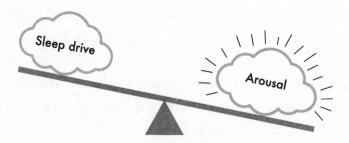

times—becomes a problem, and too much arousal is the key to your insomnia.

You're already familiar with arousal—it's what you're experiencing when your mind races at bedtime, for example, and the feeling of having restless sleep even when you do sleep. It's the feeling of being wide awake even when you're exhausted, and what keeps you tossing after waking at 3:00 A.M. These experiences are not illusions. They are actually reflected in the brain activity of people with insomnia.

Eric Nofzinger and colleagues published the definitive functional brain imaging study on this topic in 2004.* They brought twenty participants into their sleep lab for three overnights—seven had chronic insomnia and thirteen had no sleep problems. All night, the researchers measured the participants' brain waves to get an accurate picture of their sleep. They also imaged participants' brain metabolism (basically, how much fuel the brain was using) during their sleep, and again the next morning. What they found was fascinating.

First, the two groups had remarkably similar sleep. The amount of time it took them to fall asleep, for example, was only four minutes different. The percentages of light versus deep versus REM sleep, as well as total sleep duration, were statistically identical between groups too.

---

* Eric A. Nofzinger, Daniel J. Buysse, Anne Germain, Julie C. Price, Jean M. Miewald, and Ba J. David Kupfer, "Functional Neuroimaging Evidence for Hyperarousal in Insomnia," *American Journal of Psychiatry* 161, no. 11 (2004): 2126–29. http://ajp.psychiatryonline.org.

However, that didn't mean the nighttime *experience* of the groups was the same. The insomnia group's brains showed overall higher glucose metabolism at night—their brains were working *harder*, being more *aroused*. Remarkably, their brains continued to work harder during the day too. **All of this shows that people with insomnia have brains that are hyperaroused, during both the day and night, even when their actual sleep parameters seem healthy from the outside.**

This is why you feel so damn *tired* (your brain's been overworking) but you still feel like you can't sleep (your brain is still hyperaroused).

Hyperarousal is also one of the reasons why people with insomnia often don't *feel* like they're sleeping even as their brains are going through the motions of sleep. Liwen, a former patient of mine, was an intelligent and level-headed woman. She thought she was losing her mind because there were nights when she honestly felt like she didn't sleep *at all,* but her wife told her she definitely slept for at least a few hours because she was snoring and didn't stir even when her name was called. Liwen didn't believe her partner until she took a video of her literally drooling on the pillow in the middle of the night—she had even turned on the light to take the video, an event Liwen did not remember at all the next morning. But she was not losing her mind. Her experience of *sleep misperception* is actually very common for people with insomnia.* Once she began to decrease her daytime and nighttime arousal, she began to sleep more soundly, and to actually enjoy the sleep her brain was producing.

So how did arousal get so out of hand in the first place? See if this list of modern day "tigers" resonates with you:

- Chronic stress
- Worry and rumination

---

* Alison G. Harvey and Nicole K.Y. Tang, "(Mis)Perception of Sleep in Insomnia: A Puzzle and a Resolution," *Psychological Bulletin* 138, no. 1 (2012): 77–101. https://doi.org/10.1037/a0025730.

- Creative excitement
- Indignation for social injustice
- Anticipation of early morning flights (or interviews, first days of school, etc.)
- Existential dread
- Frustration about sleeplessness
- Uncertainty about whether that mole looks bigger or not than it did last year

The list could go on, as there are endless ways to get worked up, in both positive and negative ways. But no matter the source of your arousal, having too much overrides your sleep drive at night, making it hard to fall asleep or stay asleep. The tricky part is you can't fight fire with fire. **If you're holding too much arousal, trying to brute force your way to sleep is like yelling at an anxious person to "just relax, goddammit!"** It backfires.

Why can't we brute force relaxation? One of the main reasons is that we often misunderstand where arousal comes from and how it works. To help you understand it in the context of insomnia, I like to chunk the many sources of it into three categories:

1. **Conditioned arousal:** Our brains are so good at putting two and two together that we can condition ourselves to experience arousal in bed simply by repeatedly being awake (and frustrated, anxious, etc.) in bed. This is the drooling dog phenomenon we'll focus on later in this chapter.

2. **Circadian arousal:** "Circadian" refers to our internal clocks, which are crucial for keeping the complicated machinery of our bodies/brains running well. Part of the clock's job is to make us alert during the day, when we need to be awake. If your clock is confused about when exactly "day" is, it will make you alert when you don't want to be (i.e., nighttime,

wee hours of the morning). We'll delve more deeply into this in later chapters.

3. **Other arousal:** Everything else, from excitement to caffeine to stress, falls into this category. The rest of the book will help you with this broad category. Spoiler: it has to do with your daytime approach to rest, fun, thoughts, stress, relationships, your body, and most of all, the fact that you have insomnia.

Good news: if you're doing sleep consolidation from chapter 4, you're already learning to decrease all three of these arousal categories! As the scale tips in favor of sleep drive, it automatically eases up on arousal on the other side. Keep up the good work.

But let's help that scale tip even more—let's work on conditioned arousal this week. It gets its own chapter because it's so powerful and so universal for people with insomnia that we can't really move forward without addressing it first. You know you have conditioned arousal if any of these sound familiar:

- You're literally falling asleep on the couch late in the evening, but when you get yourself into bed (very quietly), it's like a light flips on in your head and suddenly you're wide-awake.
- When you wake up during the night, your brain goes from slightly awake to "let's plan our finances for the next ten years and worry about everything that might go wrong" in about three seconds flat.
- You sleep better on the couch, in the passenger seat of a car, in a hotel, or at someone else's house than in your own bed.
- You dread going to bed, or anticipate having insomnia as it gets closer to bedtime.*

---

* As one of my recent patients described it, "Sometimes I'd just stand there in the evening, looking at my bed with hatred. And I'd feel like crying."

What is this hateful force that causes these baffling and torturous insomnia experiences? Let's ease the pain by explaining it through puppies.

What Is Conditioned Arousal?

If you've ever taken a Psych 101 class, you'll have heard of Pavlov's dogs. In the 1890s, Russian physiologist Ivan Pavlov conducted a famous set of experiments studying dogs and salivation. You won't be surprised to hear that Pavlov's dogs salivated when presented with meat. Of course they did! The fun part was when he began to ring a bell every time he presented the meat, and after a few times, just the bell itself got the dogs drooling excitedly.

We're all like Pavlov's dogs, built to experience what came to be called *classical conditioning**—the process where our brains learn that if bell and meat always appear together, then we should expect meat whenever we hear a bell. For people with insomnia, the bed is the bell. The bed signals that insomnia is about to happen because the bed (and bedtime, the idea of bed, the idea of sleep, etc.) has so often gone hand-in-hand with being awake (and being frustrated, being anxious, and being anything other than asleep). In other words, all the hours you've spent tossing and turning have actually *conditioned* your brain to be awake and unhappy . . . in bed.

No wonder your brain automatically turns on when you get into bed, even if you were irresistibly sleepy just a minute ago. The brain is seeing this getting-into-bed process for the millionth time, and it's saying, "Oh yes, I know what this place is! This is where we stare at the inside of our eyelids while reviewing our to-do list. This is also where we think about

---

* Ibraheem Rehman, Navid Mahabadi, Terrence Sanvictores, and Chaudhry I. Rehman, "Classical Conditioning," *Encyclopedia of Human Behavior: Second Edition* (August 2021): 484–91. https://doi.org/10.1016/B978-0-12-375000-6.00090-2.

our ongoing insomnia problem and do a systems check on all the negative emotions—frustration, hopelessness, anger, fear, desperation—just to make sure they still work. No problem, let me get this process fired up right away!"

If you don't have trouble falling asleep but struggle to get back to sleep in the middle of the night, conditioned arousal* has its hold on you too. Your brain may associate your bedtime routine with drowsiness and relaxation, but it's been through enough 3:00 A.M. battles that it knows the drill well—as soon as there's a blink of wakefulness, dial the brain up to full alertness, and keep bringing in arousal reinforcements in the form of worries, exciting ideas, catchy songs, and rageful thoughts about how your partner woke you up with their snoring.

Sometimes, this conditioned arousal bleeds into the daytime. Even the sight of your bed or the thought of sleep might make you groan, because your body and mind have learned to resent this place so much. My former patient Frank said it best when he compared his bed to a dentist's chair. He's right! Picture someone strapped to an old-timey dentist's chair, their wild eyes scanning the tray of sharp instruments that gleam in the fluorescent light, the sound of a drill getting louder in the background. Expecting yourself to sleep well after years of conditioned arousal is like expecting a root canal patient to sleep well right now.

And what a tragic thing it is to lose the safe haven of your bed! If you don't find the refuge of sweet sleepiness in bed, and instead find phantom battles simply because so many have been fought there, of course you're tired and crabby during the day. It's exhausting to never put down your guard.

Let's learn to be *sleepy* in bed again. This is the second major strat-

---

* M. L. Perlis, D. E. Giles, W. B. Mendelson, R. R. Bootzin, and J. K. Wyatt, "Psychophysiological Insomnia: The Behavioural Model and a Neurocognitive Perspective," *Journal of Sleep Research* 6, no. 3 (1997): 179–88. https://doi.org/10.1046/J.1365-2869.1997.00045.X.

egy, after sleep consolidation (see chapter 4), we can use to reset our relationship with sleep. We've already started by feeding sleep what it needs—more sleep drive. Now let's help it feel safe and relaxed in the place where we're inviting it to spend time with us.

How to Unlearn Conditioned Arousal

To learn to be sleepy in bed, we simply have to sleep in bed—and not do much else there. In other words, if we save the bed just for sleeping, and take other activities elsewhere, our brains will eventually be reconditioned to expect sleepiness, and only sleepiness, when we get into bed.

That means these popular in-bed activities will need a new home:

- Watching TV
- Scrolling the news or social media
- Chatting on the phone
- Playing video games
- Fighting with the partner
- Eating
- Working or studying

The first thing to change is: don't use the bed for anything other than sleeping. Move your TV out of the bedroom (you can still watch it leading up to bedtime, in another room). Do your work-from-home meetings at the kitchen counter or even in the closet, if you need privacy—just don't use your bed, or ideally your bedroom, for work. Cozy up or argue with your partner on the couch, not in the bedroom. If you need your phone in your bedroom to serve as an alarm clock or because you need to be on call for some reason, put it into do not disturb mode and place it on the other side of the room.

QUICK TIP FOR CAREGIVERS AND ON-CALL PERSONNEL

If you do need to be able to receive some alerts, such as calls from your child, updates on an elderly person in your care, or emergency alerts from work when you're on call, you can program your phone such that you only receive calls from certain phone numbers or alerts from certain apps, and the rest are screened out. This way your brain doesn't need to make any in-the-moment decisions about which alerts to heed or ignore, and you won't be worried about missing something important.

If you're thinking, "Great, I don't do any of these nonsleep things in bed . . . moving on to the next chapter." **Wait! I bet there's at least one nonsleep activity you do in bed: trying to fall asleep.**

No, trying to sleep doesn't count as sleeping. Hoping for sleep, waiting for it, chasing it, pleading with it, using breathing techniques to try to coax it, counting down the amount of time you have left to sleep tonight . . . all of these are nonsleep activities. In fact, this "trying to sleep" is the very *worst* type of activity you can do in bed. It is the one that gives you the strongest, most stubborn conditioned arousal. **This is the second, and even more important new thing to start doing: when you can't fall asleep (or fall back to sleep), get up and do something else.**

This concept is called *stimulus control** in behavioral sleep medicine lingo, but I prefer to think of it as dropping the rope. Instead of continuing to struggle in a tug-of-war that gets harder and harder to win the more you pull, how about dropping the rope and doing something more enjoyable instead? Even if you do eventually "win" this tug-of-war, it will

---

* R. R. Bootzin, "Stimulus Control Treatment for Insomnia," *Proceedings of the American Psychological Association* 7, 395–96. https://doi.org/10.1037/e465522008-198.

cost you loads of angst and earn you ever more conditioned arousal, because every moment you stay in this contest, you're teaching your brain more conditioned arousal in bed. Ironically, if you decline to play tug-of-war at all, you may feel sleepy again sooner. Even if not, you weren't going to be sleeping anyway! This way, at least you will be dismantling conditioned arousal, and you get to enjoy some extra "me" time.

Frequently Asked Questions About Conditioned Arousal

How Long Should I Wait Before Getting Out of Bed?

You don't need to pop out of bed at the first sign of consciousness. But don't wait until you're frustrated with sleeplessness. I'm not going to give you a specific number of minutes to wait before getting out of bed because I don't want you to count minutes while lying there. Besides, it's not about exactly how long you've been awake. It's more about how you feel: Are you happily drifting in half sleep, or wide awake? Are you smiling to yourself about a lingering pleasant dream, or are you resentfully reviewing how little sleep you've been getting lately? Do you feel like you're on the verge of falling asleep, or can you tell it's not going to happen? If the former, feel free to keep cozying up. If the latter, it's time to drop the rope and get out of bed.

WHAT DOES BEING "SLEEPY" FEEL LIKE AGAIN?

You may not be well acquainted with the feeling of "being on the verge of falling asleep" if you've had insomnia for a while. How can you tell whether you're feeling sleepy enough to stay in bed versus awake enough that you should get up? Here's what sleepiness feels like:

- Body feels heavy and relaxed
- Eyes feel droopy, unfocused
- Mind feels drifty, unfocused
- If you're listening to a book or podcast, your attention wanders in and out of the plot, and you're not sure you're catching it all

Here are signs that you're *not* sleepy, even if you're tired:

- Body feels restless, and you're aware of all its little sensations
- You have no trouble keeping your eyes open and focusing them enough to read
- Mind is clear and able to focus; you can follow logical trains of thought
- You're actively frustrated or anxious about sleep

What Should I Do When I Get Out of Bed?

You can do anything you'd like to. The keyword here is "like." Don't watch a boring TV show or read a boring book to try to bore yourself to sleep . . . you'll just be annoyed with wasting time and soon start fretting about insomnia again. Instead, watch the show you've been looking forward to, or read the book you can hardly put down. And don't sit quietly in the dark hoping that it will trick your brain into drowsiness . . . it won't. It'll just be another version of "trying to sleep" that pushes sleep even further away. Instead, get out the paint brushes and model train sets, try a new podcast, or do anything else that feels like a treat.*

---

* That is, as long as it's not an extremely exciting activity. I feel almost silly writing this caveat, because I doubt you're going to gamble on horse races or play violent video games at 3:00 A.M. If you're not sure whether something is too exciting, don't overthink it. Just do what you like and adjust it next time if needed.

But I've Tried This Before, and It Didn't Work.
Getting Out of Bed Just Woke Me Up Even More!

Indeed, getting out of bed may wake you up even more, but the point isn't that getting out of bed will make you sleepier, and the goal of getting out of bed isn't to put you back to sleep. Instead, the goal is to prevent your brain from learning, yet again, to associate the bed with wakefulness and effort. Even if staying in bed allows you to skim the surface of sleep a little bit more, you're just teaching your brain to do half-baked sleep in the middle of the night.

If you've tried getting out of bed when you couldn't sleep before, I'm sure it didn't immediately make a difference in your insomnia. That's because conditioned arousal takes time and consistency to un-learn. It's tough to stick with this behavior change because its benefits can be invisible and gradual, but trust that you're tapping into powerful forces here.

Plus, it's not just conditioned arousal that we're getting rid of by getting out of bed. It also has the benefit of decreasing other types of arousal: rumination, effort, frustration, desperation, worry, counting the hours until your alarm clock goes off. All of the mental activities you get up to when lying there, trying and failing to sleep, increases arousal. If you're going to be awake, you might as well be awake and enjoying yourself! So go ahead and indulge in that movie you've been wanting to watch.

Won't TV or Other Screens Be Too Stimulating?
Won't the Light Be Bad for My Sleep?

First of all, any stimulation from your TV, Kindle, or phone is likely to be a much weaker force than the stimulation from conditioned arousal (and the act of "trying to sleep"). Be pragmatic—if you're going to be awake anyway, would you rather do battle and pump adrenaline while in bed, or get a little dose of light from an enjoyable TV show? That being said, maybe don't watch a horror movie or play *Grand Theft Auto*. Purposely putting yourself into crisis mode is silly in the middle of the night.* Any other activity is allowed, as long as you're not *trying* to make sleep happen.

Second, the main concern sleep scientists have with nighttime light exposure is that blue light (i.e., short wavelength light) from screens may alter your circadian rhythms, which may, in turn, affect your sleep quality (much more on this in chapter 6). The solution here is simple: dim your screen, put on Night Shift mode, or wear blue light–blocking glasses when you're up at night. If you forget to do so, it's not a big deal. As long as you're getting lots of light exposure during the day, your internal clocks will still be able to tell the difference between day and night.

But Won't Getting Out of Bed Just Teach My Brain to Wake Up at Night?

Your brain already wakes up at night. Staying in bed doesn't prevent that. Getting out of bed doesn't either, but it teaches your brain that waking up is not scary or frustrating, which in turn teaches your brain/ body to relax, instead of going into high alert mode, when you wake during the night.

---

* Personally, during the time I wrote this book, when I had trouble sleeping, I would get up and read espionage novels or write. I enjoy both very much, so either I slept or got to enjoy extra reading/writing time—a no-lose situation.

But Getting Out of Bed Means I'll Be Missing an Opportunity to Sleep, so I'll End up Even More Sleep-Deprived!

My friend, you weren't sleeping anyway. If you were, you wouldn't be having this dilemma! And how has staying in bed *trying* to sleep worked so far? It's possible that staying in bed for an hour has sometimes (maybe even often) resulted in drifting back to sleep, but all the cumulative hours of trying, either ultimately successful or not, have fanned the flame of your chronic insomnia week after week, year after year.

And remember, insomnia and sleep deprivation are not the same thing. If what's keeping you up is an internal force (e.g., racing mind), and not an external force (e.g., ongoing fireworks outside your window), it means you're probably not sleep-deprived. If you were, you'd have the opposite problem from insomnia! You'd be falling asleep when you don't want to, instead of not being able to sleep when you do.

When Should I Get Back into Bed to Try Again?

Never. You're never going to bed to *try* to sleep. Remember, sleep is an involuntary process that you can, at most, *allow* to happen. It's not one you can *make* happen. When you fully accept this truth, you'll know when to get back into bed (hint: it's when you're sleepy).

What If I Don't Have Anywhere Else to Go, or Physically Can't Leave the Bedroom?

You may very well have space restrictions in your home, especially if you live in a studio apartment, share living space with roommates, or have more people in the household than there are private rooms. Or you might have mobility restrictions that make it risky or difficult for you to leave the bed/bedroom unassisted.

If, for whatever reason, you cannot leave your bed/bedroom at night, don't worry—you can still unlearn conditioned arousal! The key is to change the context between sleeping mode and awake mode. When you can't fall asleep, don't lie in the same position in the dark and continue to let your mind race. When you do this, you're staying in sleeping mode without sleep, which increases conditioned arousal. Instead, you can switch to awake mode by turning on a light, sitting in an armchair, scooting over to the foot of the bed, getting above the covers, or doing an enjoyable activity (reading, watching a movie, etc.). The most important thing to avoid doing in bed is *trying* to sleep. So if you're stuck in your bed/bedroom overnight, have a fun book at the ready to steer you away from that temptation.

What About Sex in Bed?

Please have sex anytime and anywhere in your home you'd like. No need to abstain from sex in the bedroom, because your conditioned arousal is, sadly, not related to *that* kind of arousal.*

What About Reading in Bed?

Much earlier in my behavioral sleep medicine career I used to brandish my hickory stick and say, "Nope, you have to read somewhere else. Only sleep is allowed in bed." But this is ridiculous. If you're reading something boring specifically to trick your brain into falling asleep, cut it out. You're

---

* However, if this presents a good excuse to try something new, you can tell yourself that you're supposed to save the bed for sleeping only, so you'll have to try making love on the kitchen counter instead. Who knew that this book could also reignite your sex life?

trying too hard. But if you're reading something for fun, and it's simply a pleasant activity for you at bedtime, by all means, enjoy! Don't do it for hours, because then you'd be getting into conditioned arousal territory. But something like fifteen to thirty minutes of bedtime reading sounds lovely. Over time, bedtime reading may even turn into a sleepy cue for you.

Do I Need to Get Out of Bed When I Can't Sleep . . . Forever?

There will come a time when this question doesn't even matter, because it will be pretty rare for you to spend a big chunk of time awake during the night, and when you do, it won't feel so bad. At that time, perhaps only weeks in the future, it's still wise to follow the general philosophy of, "Don't spend a lot of time awake in bed." But it won't be catastrophic if you just don't feel like getting up. For now, earn your right to break the rule by following it consistently—the more you do so, the more quickly you'll lose your conditioned arousal.

Continuing Your Big Reset

Let's take a break from conditioned arousal to check in on how the overall Big Reset is going. If you've been working on sleep consolidation from chapter 4 for at least one week, and you've been diligently keeping your daily sleep logs (ideally using the Consensus Sleep Diary app or CBT-I Coach app), you're well on your way to the Big Reset! You may even be ready to tweak your time-in-bed window. If you haven't read chapter 4 yet, please interrupt reading this and return to chapter 4. Moving forward with the Hello Sleep program without the foundation from chapters 4 and 5 together would be like building a balcony without a first floor. Let's assess how last week went, and then talk about how to move forward with your new time-in-bed window.

1. How Is Sleep Consolidation Going?

Assess your progress by looking at your sleep logs. Note these variables:

- **Sleep efficiency:** Hopefully this is higher and closer to the 85 percent to 95 percent range we're aiming for. Don't fret if you've been faithful to the Hello Sleep program and your sleep efficiency is not there yet. It often takes a couple of weeks for your brain to fully catch up to what we're doing.
- **Total time in bed:** This should be very close to what you calculated to be your time-in-bed window in chapter 4. If it's significantly longer, that means you went to bed earlier than you were supposed to, or stayed in bed later than you were supposed to.
- **Time to fall asleep:** Was this shorter? Longer? About the same? No need to judge—just simply notice any patterns. If it took less time to fall asleep than previous weeks, might it be because you had more sleep drive saved up at bedtime? If it took longer to fall asleep, it could be totally unremarkable if it wasn't too long (about thirty minutes is pretty normal), or it could have been a fluke, or your brain was still working on catching up with what we've been doing. All scenarios are normal at this stage.
- **Time awake in the middle of the night:** Ditto above!
- **Total sleep time:** This is the least important variable at this time. It could be longer, shorter, or the same as before—any of these scenarios would be unremarkable. This is usually the last variable to change, and also the least stable and least meaningful for your healthy relationship with sleep. So, don't worry about this one right now.

2. Problem-Solve Hiccups with Sleep Consolidation

If you did not stick to the sleep consolidation instructions (e.g., your past week's average total time in bed was significantly longer than what it should have been, or you often went to bed earlier than your earliest allowed bedtime), you would be in good company. Many people have trouble with it, especially in the first week. There might be a few issues, such as:

Misunderstanding Instructions

This part of sleep therapy can be confusing, especially if you don't have a live person walking you through step-by-step. Reread chapter 4 and make sure you're using the Consensus Sleep Diary app or CBT-I Coach app. There's no rush!

Running into Logistical Barriers

Perhaps it's difficult to go to bed later than you usually do because this wakes up your bed partner. Or maybe your alarm clock is not reliable, which makes you anxious. Fixes for some common barriers are:

- **Sleep separately from your bed partner if possible.** I know that many people believe that couples should sleep in the same bed and that sleeping separately indicates a problem with the relationship. This is silly. If sleeping apart allows you to have more freedom of timing, movement, and not having to worry about disturbing someone else, why not do it? Added benefits include less noise/heat disturbance for both partners, breathing less carbon dioxide, and having more "me" time. You can still cuddle, have sex, and generally enjoy each other's company before your bedtime, at which point you can move to wherever you're spending the night to sleep. This doesn't have to be your arrangement forever. Once you don't have chronic insomnia anymore, you can reassess what works best for you and your partner.

- **Use earplugs and eye masks.** Whoever is being disturbed by hubbub from the rest of the household can shut out noise and light pretty easily and cheaply. Don't be shy to use these tools.
- **Set two alarms, if needed.** If you're worried about oversleeping your alarm, set two—one for when you should get up and one for a few minutes later as an emergency backup. Maybe one is on your phone and the other is from a traditional clock. Test both alarms for reassurance.

Having Trouble with Motivation

It's totally understandable to lose steam over the course of the week, even if you started out motivated. It's common to throw in the towel, especially if you're still having long bouts of wakefulness during the night. These points might be helpful to keep in mind:

1. **It takes some time to see change.** It doesn't take that long, in the grand scheme of your experience of insomnia, but it still takes a couple of weeks or more to see improvement. This can be frustrating. Hang in there and think of these weeks as an investment in a lifetime of having a good relationship with sleep, a relationship you intimately experience for one-quarter or more of your entire time on Earth.

2. **We're aiming for better quality first. Quantity will follow.** It might be frustrating to see yourself not sleeping any more than before, or even that you're getting less total sleep. This is normal during the Big Reset phase. That's because quantity can only be built on the foundation of quality. That's why we're teaching the brain to sleep *more efficiently* first before we can expect it to sleep longer.

3. **Remind yourself of why you're doing this.** If change is too
hard now, when will be the right time? This is an honest question. Perhaps it is not a good time to work on your relationship
with sleep right now. Perhaps your problem with sleep is not
actually severe enough to make this effort worth it. All of these
would be valid reasons to stop! You can still peruse the rest of
this book casually, without the pressure of doing the work. Just
give yourself a threshold for when things are bad enough that
it's worth trying again (e.g., "When I struggle with sleep more
than four nights per week," or "When it starts to negatively
affect my parenting"). There's no rush.

3. Update Your Time-in-Bed Window

Onward! Now you're in your second week of the Big Reset. Time to
tweak your time-in-bed window accordingly. Here's how:

- Note your past week's average sleep efficiency.
- **If it's above 90 percent, you get to have more time in bed this
  upcoming week.** Simply increase your previous time-in-bed
  window by fifteen to thirty minutes. This means you can either
  go to bed fifteen to thirty minutes earlier, or get up fifteen to
  thirty minutes later, or split the difference however you'd like.
  Remember to stick with the *same* rise time every day throughout the week, even if it's different from last week's.
- **If it's between 85 and 90 percent, let's hold steady with the
  schedule you've got from chapter 4.** Give it another week,
  along with new instructions for decreasing conditioned arousal,
  and we'll really cement that good sleep efficiency.
- **If it's lower than 85 percent, see the problem-solving tips
  above to see what you might need to do differently.** You can

either hold steady with the schedule you've got from chapter 4, or redo the time-in-bed window calculations from chapter 4 using your most recent two weeks of sleep log data. It may also just take another week or so for your brain to catch up to the sleep consolidation program.

What to Do This Upcoming Week

You're going to continue with the Big Reset, but now with two big components: sleep consolidation and decreasing conditioned arousal. All together, your instructions include:

1. Get up at your regular rise time every day: _____ [insert new rise time]

2. Don't go to bed until your earliest allowed bedtime:_____ [insert new bedtime calculated above], or until you're sleepy, whichever is *later*.

3. Don't nap or "make up" for a bad night by sleeping in or going to bed early. In other words, no matter how your sleep goes, you are not allowed in bed until your bedtime, and you must be up by your rise time. Brief naps (give or take twenty minutes) are allowed for safety.

4. Don't do anything in bed other than sleeping. However, sex and bedtime reading for fun are allowed.

5. If you can't fall asleep (or can't fall back to sleep), get out of bed and do something for fun. Do not stay in bed or *try* to fall asleep.

BOTTOM LINE

- Arousal works against sleep drive. It refers to your body or mind being revved up.
- People with insomnia experience hyperarousal, which we can see in their brain activity at night and during the day.
- There are many possible sources of arousal, but we want to start working on conditioned arousal first because it's such a big piece of the insomnia puzzle.
- Conditioned arousal is when your brain has learned to automatically become awake in bed, because you've spent so much time being awake in bed in the past. This makes your bed into a not-sleepy place.
- To reverse conditioned arousal
  » don't use the bed for anything other than sleeping (it's fine to make exceptions for sex and brief reading); and
  » when you can't fall asleep (or fall back to sleep), get up and do something else. The point is not that this will put you back to sleep, but that, over time, it will decrease conditioned arousal. A bonus benefit is that you'll enjoy your wakeful time more.
- This week, you will continue your Big Reset by recalculating your time-in-bed window based on last week's sleep log data. You will also begin to reverse conditioned arousal.
- Make sure to keep doing your sleep logs every day!

6

Let There Be Light

The Real Answers to Fatigue (Hint: It's Not More Sleep)

A few weeks into sleep therapy, I noticed that Chris's sleep looked a lot better by the numbers: he was consistently taking ten to fifteen minutes to fall asleep, and was only awake for twenty minutes on average during the night. This was a drastic change from before, when he'd be awake for one to two hours on most nights. Great work, Chris! But there was one puzzling thing—he still rated his sleep as "Poor" each morning. When I asked about this, Chris explained that he figured his sleep was bad because he still felt tired during the day. "I'm dragging my feet through mud in the morning, and I feel exhausted by afternoon. If only I could feel less tired, I'd feel great about my sleep!"

I bet you're tired of being tired.

Fatigue—the experience of feeling tired, exhausted, foggy, spent, or like you're dragging—is the most common symptom of insomnia. People with insomnia struggle with fatigue more than people with any other sleep disorder.* That translates to millions of people who can relate to you and Chris. These legions of tired-but-wired zombies are so desperate to feel more energetic during the day that they have contributed to Starbucks being a twenty-billion-dollar business. And if I had a dollar for every insomnia patient who's told me something along the lines of, "If only I could get more sleep, I wouldn't be so exhausted all the time" . . . well, I still wouldn't be *rich*, but I'd be shopping in the organic section of Whole Foods.

But what if the whole premise of this wish is based on a faulty assumption? What if it's not "lack of sleep" that's causing you to feel tired? Right now, most people with insomnia assume this is how it goes:

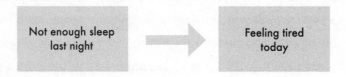

But I'm here to pitch you a new idea, one that's more supported by scientific evidence *and* more helpful for alleviating your fatigue:

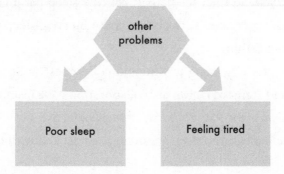

Notice that in this second diagram, poor sleep is not *causing* the fatigue. Both are caused by other problems. I know that sounds vague right now,

---

* Gentle reminder that fatigue (feeling tired) is *not* the same as sleepiness. Sleepy is when you're about to fall asleep. Tired is everything else.

but by the end of this chapter you'll know exactly what those problems are. First, let me show you why the first diagram (where "not enough sleep" directly causes "feeling tired") is *incorrect*. In fact, this worldview is not only incorrect, but is damaging, because when you hold on to that belief, you're missing out on the real solutions to fatigue *and* straining your relationship with sleep by placing unfair blame and pressure on it.

Objective Sleep Parameters Don't Predict Fatigue

Sleep is hard to measure. You can ask someone to tell you how much they slept last night—the answers reflect a person's *subjective* sleep, or their own perception and memory of it. But we've already talked about how subjective sleep is not always accurate, especially for people with insomnia. The more *objective* approach for measuring sleep is via polysomnography, or PSG (see page 42). It's the most accurate way to measure a person's sleep, and we do it in real time, getting second-by-second outputs.

All of this is to say that when we ask whether sleep truly influences our daytime functioning, the best way to find out is to measure people's sleep with PSG and then see if their *objective* sleep parameters predict their daytime experience. **It turns out that objective sleep parameters do *not* predict fatigue.**

In a 2019 study by Seog Ju Kim and colleagues* (a Sungkyunkwan University and Stanford University collaboration), 598 insomnia patients completed overnight PSG to measure their objective sleep, and *none* of the objectively measured sleep parameters correlated with fatigue:

- Total sleep duration
- Sleep efficiency

* Seog Ju Kim, Somin Kim, Sehyun Jeon, Eileen B. Leary, Fiona Barwick, and Emmanuel Mignot, "Factors Associated with Fatigue in Patients with Insomnia," *Journal of Psychiatric Research* 117, (October 2019): 24–30. https://doi.org/10.1016/j.jpsychires.2019.06.021.

- Wake after sleep onset (i.e., total time awake during the night)
- Percentage of light, deep, or REM sleep

That's right, the things that seem most obviously linked to fatigue . . . are not. What if this was a one-night fluke (for almost six hundred people)? A Canadian study by Fortier-Brochu and colleagues* kept participants with insomnia for *three* nights of PSG, and found the same thing: the amount of sleep on these three nights did *not* predict fatigue levels. In fact, when both studies zoomed out and asked for people's habitual sleep duration (i.e., how much sleep they usually got), they found that the participants with *longer* habitual sleep duration had *more* fatigue.

This doesn't necessarily mean that if you sleep more you will be more tired. The direction of cause and effect is unclear in this particular finding, and most likely it reflects a common cause that underlies *both* the longer habitual sleep duration *and* the fatigue—perhaps medical illness or depression. But for now, what we can clearly see from these studies is this: **when we measure real sleep, without bias, sleep duration is *not* associated with fatigue levels.**

Am I Just Imagining That I'm More Tired After Worse Nights?

No. Your experience of fatigue is very real. Why, then, is there this seemingly impossible contradiction between the science, which shows that sleep duration is not related to fatigue, and your experience, which surely shows that you feel more tired after sleepless nights?

---

* Émilie Fortier-Brochu, Simon Beaulieu-Bonneau, Hans Ivers, and Charles M. Morin, "Relations between Sleep, Fatigue, and Health-Related Quality of Life in Individuals with Insomnia," *Journal of Psychosomatic Research* 69, no. 5 (2010): 475–83. https://doi.org/10.1016/j.jpsychores.2010.05.005.

1. Hyperarousal Does Lead to More Fatigue

In chapter 5, we first introduced the concept of hyperarousal: when your body or brain is too revved up. I told you about the landmark brain imaging study by Nofzinger and colleagues that showed people with insomnia had higher brain metabolism during the night than healthy sleepers. Even though the two groups had the *same amount of sleep*, the insomnia group's brains were working harder at night—they were hyperaroused. And of course, having hyperarousal *is* more fatiguing than not, just like walking uphill is more fatiguing than walking on a flat surface. While your exhaustion may not necessarily be due to how little or much you slept last night, it may very well be due to you having hyperarousal.

2. Misperception of Sleep May Lead to More Fatigue

This point is related to hyperarousal too. Remember in chapter 2 when I introduced the idea of sleep misperception—the experience of feeling like one slept less than one actually did, almost universal among people with insomnia? This is due to hyperarousal, which makes your brain perceive Stage 2 sleep as not sleeping, even though Stage 2 is real sleep, which is supposed to take up about 50 percent of the night. This finding is not in the headlines, but I noticed that in the Fortier-Brochu study, insomniacs with severe fatigue were also the ones who most underestimated their sleep duration, whereas those with less fatigue had less sleep misperception. In fact, some of those with the objectively worst sleep even overestimated their sleep duration and ended up with only mild fatigue. This shows that *subjective perception* of sleep predicts fatigue much more than actual sleep duration.

3. Inconsistent Sleep Leads to More Fatigue

People with insomnia are often surprised to see that, according to their sleep logs, the average nightly sleep duration is longer than they thought. This is understandable because our memory tends to be skewed by the worst nights. But getting a consistent six and a half hours each night, every night, is very different from sometimes getting eight and a half hours and sometimes four and a half hours, and if you have insomnia, you're more likely to experience the latter scenario. A University of Toronto study by Harris and colleagues* found that this night-to-night variation around your personal average does predict fatigue after the worst nights. But they also found that comparing between people, whether someone's average is five hours a night or eight hours a night, did not predict which person was more tired overall. This means it's not the total *amount* of sleep that matters. It's the consistency.

4. There's Often Circular Logic and Self-Fulfilling Prophecies When It Comes to Sleep and Fatigue

If your ironclad belief is that being tired during the day is due to not sleeping enough, and you're currently feeling tired, you will infer that you didn't sleep enough last night. And when someone asks what not getting enough sleep does to you, you'd say, "It makes me tired the next day."

The Harris study investigated thinking styles that drive the relationship between insomnia severity and fatigue severity. They found that people with more severe insomnia tend to ruminate more about fatigue (e.g., often think about how tired they feel, how they don't have the energy to get

---

* Andrea L. Harris, Nicole E. Carmona, Taryn G. Moss, and Colleen E. Carney, "Testing the Contiguity of the Sleep and Fatigue Relationship: A Daily Diary Study," *Sleep* 44, no. 5 (2021). https://doi.org/10.1093/SLEEP/ZSAA252.

through the day, or otherwise dwell on fatigue) and to hold "dysfunctional beliefs" about sleep (e.g., having insomnia is catastrophic). In turn, **ruminating about fatigue and having unhelpful sleep beliefs led to more fatigue.** This makes sense because fretting about fatigue and sleep problems is exhausting! And frequently shining a spotlight on how tired you feel gives fatigue an outsized presence in your life, magnifying how bad it feels, and preventing you from having more fun, which makes you feel worse about your sleep, which makes you more hyperaroused, which makes your sleep worse. Prophecy fulfilled.

What the Heck Is Making Me So Tired Then?

Now we know that "other problems" include hyperarousal, sleep misperception, inconsistent sleep, and the way we think about sleep/fatigue. All these issues give us insomnia at night and fatigue during the day. The good news is that you've already begun to address them if you're doing the Hello Sleep program (e.g., working on sleep consolidation and reversing conditioned arousal). Now, let's turn our attention to some more of these "other problems" that make us tired.

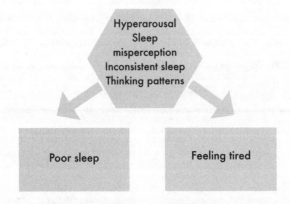

Understand that there are many, many potential sources of fatigue. Here's a short list of suspects, in no particular order:

- Circadian dysregulation
- Sedentariness
- Depression
- Occupational or family stress
- Stress from racism and other discrimination
- Being female*
- High BMI
- Inflammation
- Anemia
- Hormonal changes
- Menopause, pregnancy, childbirth (and the months that follow)
- Illness (diabetes, cancer, thyroid disease, autoimmune disease, etc.)
- Medical treatment (chemotherapy, dialysis, etc.)
- Medication side effect (including sleep medications)
- Pain or injury
- Trauma, posttraumatic stress disorder (PTSD)
- Eye strain
- Poor nutrition
- Substance use (including tobacco, alcohol, caffeine)

If any of these apply to you, you may have been unfair to blame sleep for all of your tiredness. If multiple suspects apply to you, sleep is almost certainly not the prime culprit nor the true answer to your fatigue. Each of the above deserves its own book (or library), and most are outside the scope of our work here. Part IV of this book will discuss topics like PTSD, menopause, and pain. For now, let's focus on just three of the most common sources of fatigue.

---

* There's not enough research to show whether "being female" is associated with more fatigue because of biological sex differences, or because women experience sexism, perform unpaid labor, and do more care-taking. Researchers have left me a bit salty by just leaving it at "being female," as if that were a fatigue-inducing medical condition in itself.

Circadian Dysregulation

Remember in chapter 1 when we talked about circadian rhythms? Quick refresher: every biological process in the body follows a roughly twenty-four-hour pattern, including when we sleep and when we wake. This complex system is directed by the suprachiasmatic nucleus (SCN), which is like a maestro in your brain that makes sure a big orchestra of separate instruments all play in sync and on time. Your SCN is happiest when it knows what time it is and is therefore able to keep everything, including your sleep-wake rhythm, on time.

"Circadian dysregulation" is a catch-all term to describe any situation where your SCN is confused about what time it is outside, or how long a day lasts. This is quite common, and it happens when you are:*

- Doing night- or rotating-shift work
- Traveling across time zones
- Waking up or falling asleep at inconsistent times across the week
- Eating meals at irregular or unconventional times
- Napping haphazardly at random times
- Living as a biologically hardwired night owl in a morning people's world (or vice versa)
- Spending a lot of time indoors during the day
- Being very sedentary during the day

When your SCN is confused by these circumstances, it has a hard time making you sleepy at night, *and* it has a hard time making you alert and energetic during the day. These clock confusion and cave-dwelling

---

* It's important to note that most of these items are much more common among people with racial/ethnic minority backgrounds and those with a low income. This is a big part of why there are sleep health disparities, where minority and underprivileged groups have higher rates of sleep problems, which in turn contributes to higher rates of other physical and mental health problems.

effects are huge but often overlooked contributors to fatigue. Many of my patients—especially ones who don't identify as natural morning people—have been shocked by how much more energetic they felt once they literally brightened their days and got their circadian systems back on track.

LET THERE BE LIGHT!

The Formula for a Happy, Healthy Circadian System

Our prehistoric ancestors got lots of light exposure during the day and virtually none at night, other than warm-colored campfire light that didn't stimulate the SCN. Nowadays, with our chronically dim daytimes and well-lit night times, light therapy* can help to nudge our prehistoric brains and improve many aspects of sleep-wake health, including fatigue. To get the most out of this (mostly) free resource:

1. **Get lots of bright light during the day, especially first thing in the morning.** This does not mean sitting in a room with the lights on—artificial lights do not have quite the same beneficial effects as sunlight. Ideally, you want to spend time outside. A study of more than four hundred thousand people in the United Kingdom found that the more time people spent outside, the better they slept, the less fatigue they felt, and the better their mood was.[†] Getting light exposure early in the day and getting a big dose (e.g., being in direct sunlight for at least a few minutes at some point during the day) are especially beneficial for sleep! This ac-

* Annette van Maanen, Anne Marie Meijer, Kristiaan B. van der Heijden, and Frans J. Oort, "The Effects of Light Therapy on Sleep Problems: A Systematic Review and Meta-Analysis," *Sleep Medicine Reviews* 29 (October 2016): 52–62. https://doi.org/10.1016/J.SMRV.2015.08.009.

† Angus C. Burns, Richa Saxena, Céline Vetter, Andrew J. K. Phillips, Jacqueline M. Lane, and Sean W. Cain, "Time Spent in Outdoor Light Is Associated with Mood, Sleep, and Circadian Rhythm-Related Outcomes: A Cross-Sectional and Longitudinal Study in over 400,000 UK Biobank Participants," *Journal of Affective Disorders* 295 (January 2021): 347–52. https://doi.org/10.1016/J.JAD.2021.08.056.

tually leads to more deep sleep later that night.* If you don't get at least an hour total of outdoor time per day, and especially if you don't live/work in a very bright space with big windows, use a blue light–enriched light box or light goggles for about twenty minutes in the morning.

2. **Keep things dim and low-key in the evenings.** People who live in neighborhoods that have bright outdoor artificial lights on at night tend to have less and worse quality sleep.† Some of this you cannot control, but some you can, such as keeping your own indoor lights dim at night. Generally, I recommend dimming things down a couple of hours before your usual bedtime. For example, put your phone and tablet on Night Shift mode, and switch from broad-spectrum overhead lights to more orangey lamps, or wear blue light–blocking glasses. The idea is to mimic having only campfires, instead of the sun, in your evening environment. I especially recommend this for people with very late chronotypes (i.e., night owls).

3. **Day versus night contrast is key.** Don't fret if you like to watch TV or use your tablet in the evenings. You don't have to quit screens entirely after sunset. They actually don't affect your nighttime melatonin or sleepiness if you've gotten lots of bright light exposure during the day. In fact, the brighter your days, the less nighttime light will affect you.‡ That's because the contrast between day and night is what tells your brain the difference. The

---

* Emma J. Wams, Tom Woelders, Irene Marring, Laura Van Rosmalen, Domien G. M. Beersma, Marijke C. M. Gordijn, and Roelof A. Hut, "Linking Light Exposure and Subsequent Sleep: A Field Polysomnography Study in Humans," *Sleep* 40, no. 12 (2017). https://doi.org/10.1093/SLEEP/ZSX165.

† Maurice M. Ohayon, and Cristina Milesi, "Artificial Outdoor Nighttime Lights Associate with Altered Sleep Behavior in the American General Population," *Sleep* 39, no. 6 (2016): 1311–20. https://doi.org/10.5665/SLEEP.5860.

‡ Tomoaki Kozaki, Ayaka Kubokawa, Ryunosuke Taketomi, and Keisuke Hatae, "Effects of Day-Time Exposure to Different Light Intensities on Light-Induced Melatonin Suppression at Night," *Journal of Physiological Anthropology* 34, no. 1 (2015): 1–5. https://doi.org/10.1186/S40101-015-0067-1/FIGURES/4.

most important thing is still to get lots of bright light during the day. If you work in a dim environment all day long, without the opportunity to go outside or use a light box, minimize screens or wear blue light–blocking glasses in the evening.

Bonus: Get up at the same time every morning and eat regular meals. Choose a rise time that is feasible to keep throughout the week (and get creative about your morning routine to buy yourself a later rise time if you'd like to sleep later). Don't skip breakfast. Don't skip lunch. Have dinner at about the same time every day. The most important thing is to let your body know when morning begins by getting out of bed and eating breakfast.

Sedentariness

In a classic 1987 study,* Robert Thayer gave people either a candy bar or told them to take a ten-minute walk, and then asked them to keep track of how energetic, tired, and tense they felt for the next two hours. Who would you guess felt better? In our daily lives, we may indeed reach for a sugary snack to get a boost of "energy," but it turns out that the people who ate the snack felt more tense and tired. The people who went for a walk instead felt more energized and less tired.

And it's not necessarily the sugar that caused tension and fatigue. It may very well be that the snackers simply missed out on the benefits of walking. For decades, studies have shown that being sedentary is associated with more fatigue, and that increasing physical activity leads to feeling more energized.†

---

* Robert E. Thayer, "Energy, Tiredness, and Tension Effects of a Sugar Snack Versus Moderate Exercise," *Journal of Personality and Social Psychology* 52, no. 1 (1987): 119–25. https://doi.org/10.1037/0022-3514.52.1.119.

† Laura D. Ellingson, Alexa E. Kuffel, Nathan J. Vack, and Dane B. Cook, "Active and Sedentary Behaviors

This doesn't mean you have to take up marathon running or Cross-Fit. Multiple studies have shown that low- to moderate-intensity exercise is best for increasing vigor and decreasing fatigue. For example, a 2016 study* found that previously sedentary college students felt less tired (including less "emotionally exhausted") after low-intensity walking/running (i.e., low-key enough that they could hold a conversation throughout the jog) three times per week for several weeks. They were specifically told *not* to aim for running as fast or as long as possible, but rather to focus on "feeling good." And don't worry if you're not a twenty-year-old spring chicken like the participants in this study. Other studies of middle-aged and older adults have found similar results.

LET THERE BE MOVEMENT!

Let's Plan Some Physical Activity

1. Choose three days of the week when you'd like to get active: _____, _____, and _____

2. Choose a fun activity to do. (Bonus points if it's outdoors or social!)

- Walking
- Jogging
- Bicycling
- Gardening
- Swimming
- Dancing
- Yoga or Tai Chi

Influence Feelings of Energy and Fatigue in Women," *Medicine and Science in Sports and Exercise* 46, no. 1 (2014): 192–200. https://doi.org/10.1249/MSS.0B013E3182A036AB.

* Juriena D. de Vries, Madelon L. M. van Hooff, Sabine A. E. Geurts, and Michiel A. J. Kompier, "Exercise as an Intervention to Reduce Study-Related Fatigue among University Students: A Two-Arm Parallel Randomized Controlled Trial," *PloS One* 11, no. 3 (2016). https://doi.org/10.1371/JOURNAL.PONE.0152137.

- Babysitting
- Assembling IKEA furniture
- Shopping
- Other: _____
- Other: _____

3. Set a reminder on your phone for your three activities or call a friend *right now* to schedule an activity date for the upcoming week. Put a sticky note reminder on your fridge or bathroom mirror.

4. Optional: Buy yourself a sticker chart and some stickers so you can keep track of your physical activity progress. There's no reason why only kids get to have fun stickers.

Depression

Even if you don't have depression, read this. I had one patient, who was an older gentleman, retired and widowed, but surrounded by loving grandkids and perpetually optimistic. Hugh improved his sleep quite quickly, but continued to feel very tired. After some more exploration of his day-to-day experiences, I realized that he was experiencing depression for the first time in his life, and he didn't know it. When I floated this idea to Hugh, he said, "But with all due respect, I'm not the mopey, pessimistic, woe-is-me type at all!"

But this is not what depression means. Depression is not a personality type or a worldview. It's a biological brain state, and if severe enough, a brain disease. It doesn't affect everyone the same way. For some people, their outlook on life changes, and for others, it shows up more as a physical change—the body feels heavier, slower . . . and more tired.

In the 2019 Stanford-Sungkyunkwan study, people with insomnia and severe fatigue scored nearly twice as high on depression as those with insomnia and mild fatigue. Since everybody in the study had insomnia, we know it's not so much the insomnia that mattered for how tired they were—it was depression. The relationship was even more striking in Fortier-Brochu and colleagues' Canadian study. Besides age, depression was the *only* factor that predicted fatigue levels, out of a dozen factors ranging from medical conditions to anxiety to occupation.

You may think, "But I really don't have depression!" Well, the people in that study technically didn't either. The researchers specifically excluded people with clinically diagnosable levels of depression from the study. But depression isn't black-or-white. We all have depressive symptoms sometimes. They can include:

- Feeling unmotivated
- Feeling down, blue, or like things are pointless
- Feeling irritable
- Feeling lonely
- Having low confidence or optimism
- Having a hard time recovering from setbacks
- Having less interest in pleasurable activities
- Feeling more guilt or resentment
- Feeling less social or creative
- Having less interest in sex
- Having a low appetite or overeating
- Having trouble concentrating or making decisions
- Sleeping less than usual
- Feeling more tired than usual

If you can relate to a few of these, like my patient did, you may be experiencing at least a mild level of depression, which is extremely common. It can be a normal response to shorter and more overcast days during the winter, stressful events or illness, work-related burnout or boredom, relationship difficulties, hormonal changes (including menstrual), and many other biological, psychological, environmental, and social changes. Depression can feel like a constant low simmer, or it might come in intense weeks-long bouts. If you think you may have persistent or more than mild depression, I strongly encourage you to ask your doctor for a referral to a clinical psychologist, psychiatrist, or other mental health professional who specializes in mood disorders.

Meanwhile, no matter your level of depression, there are two very effective ways to boost your mood and vitality—light* and movement.† **That's right. What you've already planned for your physical activity and bright light exposure during the day just happen to be some of the best therapy for depression too.**

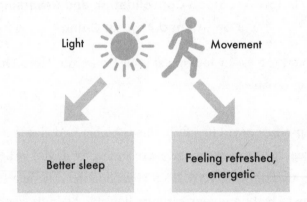

Hugh, the retired and widowed gentleman, took up a combination light-and-movement regimen. He started taking a morning walk outside. He fixed his bicycle and went on weekend rides. He volunteered to babysit the grandkids. He even picked up volunteer work at the lo-

---

* Golden, Robert N., Bradley N. Gaynes, R. David Ekstrom, Robert M. Hamer, Frederick M. Jacobsen, Trisha Suppes, Katherine L. Wisner, and Charles B. Nemeroff. "The Efficacy of Light Therapy in the Treatment of Mood Disorders: A Review and Meta-Analysis of the Evidence," *American Journal of Psychiatry* 162 (2005): 656–62. https://doi.org/10.1176/APPI.AJP.162.4.656/ASSET/IMAGES/LARGE/N93F5.JPEG.

† Schuch, Felipe B., Davy Vancampfort, Justin Richards, Simon Rosenbaum, Philip B. Ward, and Brendon Stubbs. "Exercise as a Treatment for Depression: A Meta-Analysis Adjusting for Publication Bias," *Journal of Psychiatric Research* 77 (June 2016): 42–51. https://doi.org/10.1016/J.JPSYCHIRES.2016.02.023.

cal dog shelter for some extra get-out-of-the-house time. I'm happy to report that he really blossomed after this. To his delight, he felt more energetic than he had in years, and his sleep improved even more.

Continuing Your Big Reset

This section looks similar to the end of chapter 5, but read it carefully because there are some changes specific to your current stage in the journey.

1. How Are Sleep Consolidation and Reversing Conditioned Arousal Going?

Assess your progress by looking at your Consensus Sleep Diary report. Note these variables:

- **Sleep efficiency:** Hopefully this is higher and closer to the 85 percent to 95 percent range we're aiming for. If you've been consistently following your sleep consolidation schedule (i.e., not going to bed until your earliest allowable bedtime, getting out of bed at your daily rise time) for over two consecutive weeks, you should be seeing changes in sleep efficiency.
- **Total time in bed:** This should be very close to what you calculated to be your time-in-bed window in chapter 5. If significantly longer, that means you went to bed earlier than you were supposed to, or stayed in bed later than you were supposed to.
- **Time to fall asleep:** Generally, if this is under thirty minutes on average, or under thirty minutes on the vast majority of nights, you're falling asleep like a healthy sleeper. If not, you're likely still going to bed too early; try staying up fifteen to thirty

minutes later. Also make sure you're keeping the same rise time every day!

- **Time awake in the middle of the night:** If you have no trouble falling asleep but spend significant time awake during the night, you're experiencing conditioned arousal. Do make sure you're getting out of bed during the night once you start to feel fully awake or starting to have a "racing mind."

- **Total sleep time:** This is the least important variable right now. It could be longer, shorter, or the same as before—any of these cases wouldn't be meaningful. This is the last variable to change, and also the least stable and least meaningful for your healthy relationship with sleep. So, don't worry about this one for the time being.

2. Problem-Solve Hiccups with Reversing Conditioned Arousal

Here are some common barriers to reversing conditioned arousal:

- **You can't fall asleep without the TV:** Perhaps it's been your habit to watch TV in bed for a very long time, and perhaps you even feel like it helps you to fall asleep. I'll still encourage you to watch TV in another room, or better yet, read a physical book on the couch or in bed. If this absolutely does not work for you after you give it an honest attempt for a week, go ahead and watch TV in bed, but try to dim the screen and make sure you set a sleep timer for an hour or less. If it's taking you longer than an hour of TV-watching to fall asleep, you were not ready to be in bed in the first place.

- **It's hard to get up during the night:** I know, it's *so* tempting to stay in bed, where it's cozy and where you *might* fall back asleep. But whatever amount of dozing you're able to skim during a wakeful bout in bed, if it's also accompanied by having "racing mind" or angst about sleep, it is not worth long-term conditioned arousal. If you don't feel like you're awake and angsty enough to get out of bed, and the dozing is actually restful, you're probably experiencing light sleep, and this period of time should not be counted as "awake" on your sleep log.

- **Getting up during the night makes you even more awake.** That's okay! The point isn't to create more sleepiness. The point is to avoid being awake for long periods in bed and further cementing conditioned arousal. If you feel like getting up is waking you up, take the opportunity to enjoy the extra "me" time and know that you're saving up both sleep drive and teaching your brain to be sleepy in bed.

- **It's hard to not do other activities in bed.** If you have space limitations, I can understand having a hard time saving the bed for sleeping only. Just try your best to differentiate between "sleeping" mode and "active" mode. For example, if you have to study in your bedroom because your roommates are playing loud video games in the living room, try to do it at a desk (or beanbag, armchair, floor, etc.), or if it must be on the bed, have your head at the foot of the bed. Turn on the ceiling light for active times, and switch to the bedside lamp for wind down times. Tune in to an upbeat soundtrack if you're playing with your kid in the bed, and switch to soothing music leading up to bedtime.

3. Update Your Time-in-Bed Window

Onward! Now you're in your third week of the Big Reset, and we'll tweak your time-in-bed window accordingly. Here's how:

- Note your past week's average sleep efficiency.
- **If it's above 90 percent, you get to have more time in bed this**

upcoming week. Simply increase your previous time-in-bed window by fifteen to thirty minutes. This means you can either go to bed fifteen to thirty minutes earlier, or get up fifteen to thirty minutes later, or split the difference however you'd like. Remember to stick with the *same* rise time every day throughout the week.

- **If it's between 85 percent and 90 percent, let's hold steady with the schedule you got from chapter 5.** Give it another week and see how things go when you add the daytime/evening techniques from this chapter.

- **If it's lower than 85 percent, see the problem-solving tips from chapter 5 and from pages 133–134 to see what you might need to do differently.** You'll likely want to hold steady with the schedule you got from chapter 5. Hang in there! What's two to three weeks more of bootcamp when you've already had insomnia for years?

What to Do This Upcoming Week

You're going to continue with the Big Reset, now with three major components: sleep consolidation, reversing conditioned arousal, and starting your light + movement routine. All together, your instructions include:

1. Get up at your regular rise time every day: _____ [insert new rise time].

2. Don't go to bed until your earliest allowed bedtime:_____ [insert new bedtime from calculated above], or until you're sleepy, whichever is *later*.

3. Don't "make up" for a bad night by sleeping in or going to bed early. In other words, no matter how your sleep goes, you are not allowed in bed until your bedtime, and you must be up by

your rise time. *If your sleep efficiency was above 90 percent, you're now allowed a midday twenty-minute nap if you feel sleepy.*

4. Don't do anything in bed other than sleeping. However, sex and bedtime reading for fun are allowed.

5. If you can't fall asleep (or can't fall back to sleep), get out of bed and do something for fun. Do not stay in bed or *try* to fall asleep.

6. Use your chapter 6 worksheets (see pages 125–129) to begin your light + movement routine:
   • Creating contrast between bright days and dim evenings
   • Getting active, ideally outside, during the day, 3 times per week

---

BOTTOM LINE

- Fatigue is the most common symptom of insomnia, and often the most irksome.
- Surprisingly, how much sleep you get overall is not associated with how tired you are during the day,
  » but experiencing hyperarousal during the day and night does make you tired;
  » and so does having a lot of variation in your sleep quantity/quality; and
  » misperceiving sleep and ruminating about sleep/fatigue problems (very common in insomnia) also leads to more fatigue.
- There are many possible factors contributing to daytime fatigue, including these three common ones:
  » Circadian dysregulation: Your circadian clock is confused because of inconsistent schedules or lack of daytime light exposure.
  » Sedentariness: Not having much physical activity makes us *more* tired.

» Depression: Even if you don't think you have "real" depression, symptoms of even mild depression can put a damper on our energy levels.

- Two of the most effective treatments for these fatigue factors are light and movement.
  » Light—get lots of it during the day, and much less at night; make sure the day-night contrast in your environment is as big as possible.
  » Movement—get active! Even twenty minutes of low- to moderate-intensity exercise (e.g., walking) can make a difference in your fatigue (and depression and sleep).
- This week, you will continue your Big Reset by recalculating your time-in-bed window based on last week's sleep log data. You will also continue to reverse conditioned arousal and start your light + movement routine.
- Make sure to keep doing your sleep logs every day!

The Mental Litter Box

*. . . and Other Daytime Skills for Quieting a
Racing Mind at Night*

Among people with insomnia, no experience is more universal than the "racing mind"—something that comes alive in the darkness, grows clinging tentacles, and gains such traction that no amount of pleading or threatening can save you from its grasp. This "racing mind" can include any or all types of thoughts—positive, negative, neutral, bizarre, boring, anxious, etc. But one thing everyone has in common is that they want to learn how to turn it off. If only you knew how to do this, you'd never have insomnia again, right? Is chamomile tea the secret? Slowing down your breathing? Imagining your happy place? Concentrating really hard on clearing your mind? (What other techniques have you already tried?)

No. I'm sorry—this book will not teach you to "turn off" your brain because it's impossible. It's also impossible to "clear your mind." Here, give it a try: Do not, at the risk of death, think of a pink elephant with purple polka dots. Don't do it! What happened? Well, it's similarly impossible to tell yourself, "Don't worry about that pending test result," or "Don't go over that embarrassing thing you said from ten years ago," or "Shut up, brain!"

Are we forever doomed to random and unrelenting attacks from our hyperactive brains at night because there's no off switch? Also no. **We can't brute force our brains into turning off, but we can teach them to know the difference between get-it-done mode and let-it-go mode, and to easily transition from one to the other at night without much wrangling on your part.** Specifically, there are three main ways to help your mind to "let it go" at night:

1. **Increase sleep drive.** Usually, it's not that the racing mind is keeping you awake—it's because you're awake that your mind is racing. In other words, if you're sleepy enough, there is simply no room for your mind to race because your mind is already crowded with drowsiness. You've already started to increase sleep drive through your work in chapter 4.

2. **Decrease conditioned arousal.** If your brain doesn't expect to get busy whenever you're in bed (conditioned arousal), it's much less likely for a stray thought to gather momentum and turn into a thought tornado. You've already started to decrease conditioned arousal through your work in chapter 5.

3. **Decrease other types of arousal.** This "other" arousal category is all about things that happen during our waking hours, which will be the focus of the rest of this book. In this chapter, we will start chipping away at daytime sources of arousal that are especially good at revving up your racing mind at night.

How Does Our Daytime Behavior Affect the Racing Mind at Night?

When we as a society talk about sleep, we're usually talking about nighttime—what to do to fall asleep, to stay asleep, to sleep more soundly, etc. But what happens during the day makes up more than half of the ingredients in the chronic insomnia soup. Let's expose three day-time / evening sabotages that feed nighttime insomnia:

1. Lack of daytime rest
2. Lack of daytime opportunity to "process" thoughts
3. Lack of a transition period before bedtime

Sabotage #1: Lack of Daytime Rest

As a parent and professional with too many interests, I know what it's like to be in get-it-done mode all day—planning, strategizing, learning, problem-solving, multitasking, crisis-managing. The source of your mental go, go, go might not be children or career mojo, but I bet that you often feel a fire under your butt to be productive. In fact, here's a quick thought experiment: Imagine that, starting right now, you're not allowed to do *anything* productive—not even reading this book, not even folding laundry—for a whole hour. What is your immediate emotional reaction?

If your immediate reaction is one of relief or joy, congratulations, you have not been taken hostage by grind culture.* But if you're like 90 percent of my corporate workshop attendees, you felt a little stab of anxiety or guilt. (*What do you mean, "Do nothing"? What would I do with myself?* See, there you go again—you can't let go of *doing*.)

How is this related to sleep? Well, think about our early human ancestors, whose biology we inherited. If they were doing and going all day long, what does that mean? It means there must have been a tiger stalking them, because otherwise, why wouldn't they have stopped to rest? If they finished a morning hunt and all was safe on the horizon,

---

* This refers to our capitalism-fueled culture of constant production and consumption, where every-thing's and everyone's value is benchmarked by economic output / potential.

they would lounge, nibble, make cave paintings, groom each other. What message are we, with our productivity addiction, sending to our chronically hyperaroused bodies and brains? We're saying, "There's a perpetual tiger on our tail!" And if there's a tiger on our tail, it would be literally fatal to fall asleep. Of course, your body and brain have trouble switching into let-it-go mode at night.

Now be honest with yourself—when do you rest? I mean, *truly* rest—not "veg out" in front of the TV to be passively stimulated by other people's drama, not mindlessly stress-eating potato chips between client meetings, not doing dishes while catching up on the latest political podcast. When do you actually feed your body and soul?

A QUICK WORD ABOUT TV (AND VIDEO GAMES, SOCIAL MEDIA, ETC.)

Don't get me wrong—consuming media is not all bad. I'm personally a big fan of TV and movies. I've done marathons of entire seasons—yes, plural—of *Breaking Bad* in one sitting. But this is not necessarily true rest. Ask yourself these questions:

- Am I watching my third hour of TV tonight because my mind and soul are being further rejuvenated, or am I doing it because I feel tired and bored? Am I really less tired or bored after watching several hours of TV?
- Is my video gaming interfering with my real-life relationships? Does my partner wish I spent more time with them? Does my body wish I spent more time caring for it?
- Do I feel good—physically, mentally, and spiritually—after spending an hour scrolling Twitter or TikTok or Instagram?
- Did I make a deliberate choice to watch this YouTube video, or did it just start playing after I watched the other one?

> **Challenge yourself to replace 25 percent of your passive media consumption time with simply being with yourself, and see what other feelings, thoughts, desires, and interactions arise.**

What to Do Instead

Judy, an entrepreneur and mother of three teenagers (yikes), happened to go on a girls' trip with her friends in the middle of insomnia therapy. She came back feeling puzzled, saying, "I slept *so well* when I was in Charleston with my girlfriends, but when I got back, I started having trouble again almost immediately." When I asked how she knew she slept better during her trip, she responded matter-of-factly, "Well, I felt refreshed and energetic during the day, so I must have slept better." From chapter 6, we know that her assumption is wrong—that how you slept last night is probably not the main thing that determines how you feel today. In fact, when we looked at her sleep logs, her sleep numbers (total sleep time, sleep efficiency, number of awakenings, etc.) were nearly identical between vacation nights and at-home nights. In fact, she slept a little bit less while on vacation because she had stayed up late to party with her friends.

If it wasn't sleeping more, what was making her feel so great in Charleston? It turns out that she laughed a lot with her friends, played games, listened to music, walked around the city, went on a sailboat with a handsome captain . . . all without checking her work email or putting out fires for her family. In other words, she *rested*.

True rest is rejuvenating for your body and mind. It's not goal-oriented, and often, what you have to show for it at the end isn't quantifiable. Even when we're not on a getaway vacation, we can rest. It might take the form of:

- Walking
- Daydreaming
- Reading
- Birdwatching
- Listening to music
- Playing music
- Stretching
- Knitting
- Chatting
- Bathing
- Doing nails, doing hair
- Building a birdhouse
- Cuddling
- Doodling
- Twiddling a blade of grass
- Sipping coffee on the porch
- Decorating cupcakes
- Looking through sentimental pictures

Still not sure what true rest means? Remember back to your childhood. Why did you pretend to be a pirate, or have tea parties with your dolls, or dig holes in the dirt? It wasn't because you *should*. If you ask a kid, they'd say, "I dunno. *Because.*" Whatever activity your adult self can feel that way about might just be rest.

However much resting you're doing now . . . double it, triple it. You may protest, "But I don't have time to rest! My day is already packed." I can relate to this very much, but I bet that if you get creative, you may find that you could replace your habitual post-dinner news-watching with music or stretching. Or that your kids can stand to do one fewer extracurricular activity, and you can use that drop-off/pick-up time for a walk instead. Or that you can replace one made-from-scratch dinner per week with a Costco frozen lasagna and play with your dog while the oven does the work. Whatever we prioritize, we do. **We've simply been taught to deprioritize rest, as if it's useless, empty space between "productive" pursuits. But in truth, it's the water between continents—the very thing that makes life possible.** Learn to love it and prioritize it again, even if it takes some discipline to do so at first.

Keep Calm and Take a Break! Let's Plan Some Rest:

1. Choose a five- to thirty-minute window for workdays when you will rest: _____

2. Choose a five- to thirty-minute window for nonworkdays when you will rest: _____

3. What restful activities will you do? (Try for options other than "vegging out" with the TV or scrolling through social media.)

   - _____
   - _____
   - _____
   - _____

Set a daily reminder on your phone *right now* to do them at the planned times.

FOR THOSE OF US WHO ARE "TYPE A"

If the thought of doing nothing for an hour makes you nervous, go to rest rehab for a week:

- **Schedule a one-hour rest period daily**, but treat it as a work meeting (e.g., put an event on the team calendar and mark yourself as "busy"). You can't miss it because it's a "work meeting." Nobody needs to know specifically what you're working on, but you know you'll be working on rest.

- **Set a boundary between "work time" and "off work time" in stone** (e.g., work is between 9:00 A.M. and 5:00 P.M.). Stop your phone from sending you work email notifications. Don't open your laptop during your "off" time. Twiddle your thumbs. Ride out the withdrawal symptoms.
- **Say "no" to at least one request per day**, whether in your personal or professional life. Practice how to say "no" kindly but firmly in the mirror or by typing out sample "no" emails.
- **Embrace boredom.** Get reacquainted with this feeling. Don't automatically fill it with something "productive." See what else you might drift toward as you get more bored. Doodling, perhaps, or people-watching in the park, or simply breathing.

Sabotage #2: Lack of Daytime Opportunity to "Process" Thoughts

When during a typical day do you process your thoughts? Let me rephrase: When do you reflect on important or joyful events, remember nostalgic places and times, make peace with worrisome things you can't control, daydream about fantastical futures, or let your curiosity and creativity lead you down random paths? You may well be doing this "processing" already if you routinely journal, for example, or do daily homework set by your therapist.

But I'm guessing many of you are going through the day on autopilot, pausing to be thoughtful only to the extent necessary to perform the task at hand or to plan for a future event. Or perhaps your mind is processing all the time, aimlessly running in circles . . . so a hum of background noise is in your head all day, but you're rarely indulging your most interesting or worrying thoughts with your full attention. Meanwhile, your thoughts are constantly trying to get your attention, tugging at your sleeve like children who *just* want to show you something important. You keep pushing them off and asking them to wait while you're getting distracted, until . . .

You turn out the last light and lay your head on the pillow. All is quiet. All is dark. For the first time today, there's nothing to distract you. Suddenly: *hooray!* The impatient thoughts are thrilled to finally get their turn. *It's about time! Let's release all the ideas and worries and venting and random memory replays at top speed!* And so it begins—the racing mind.

What to Do Instead

If you give yourself a proper chance to process thoughts during the day or evening, they won't be bouncing around your head at night with so much energy. **The solution is simple: make sure you have protected time during the day to give your thoughts full attention.** Some options are:

- **Keep a daily journal.** Don't expect yourself to write masterful prose, which will just make you procrastinate. Let your journal simply be a place for dumping your stream-of-consciousness (a.k.a. word vomit). Feel free to immediately burn each entry so you don't have to see how bad the writing was.
- **Engage in solo prayer.** If prayer is already part of your spiritual practice and gives you the opportunity to honestly reflect on your thoughts, fears, joys, hopes . . . do it more! Group prayer can be wonderful, but this setting doesn't always allow for full expression of your inner thoughts, so make sure you have daily solo praying too.

- **Take long walks.** Let your mind wander along with your feet. Feel free to think out loud to yourself as you walk. Make the walks longer than twenty minutes, if possible.

- **Make a mental litter box.** This one is especially good for people who are prone to worry or ruminate. If you have cats, you know that you'd better have a litter box in the house to avoid finding turds all over your furniture. Our minds are like cats—quick, entertaining, and prone to do business anywhere there isn't a designated box for it. Make a litter box for your worry-prone mind: teach it to only poop in one designated part of your day instead of dumping worry whenever and wherever it feels like. You'd be surprised how much your mind, much like a kitten, appreciates having this kind of boundary. This one doesn't work for everyone, but when it does, it's like magic. See instructions below.

HOW TO MAKE A MENTAL LITTER BOX

1. **Choose a thirty-minute block of time to set aside each day**: _____to _____A.M./P.M. If it's hard to squeeze out this much uninterrupted time every day, feel free to overlap it with an autopilot type of activity (e.g., afternoon commute, doing dishes).

2. **During this mental litter box half hour, worry as much as possible.** Don't try to talk yourself out of worries or "be positive." Let your worrying hair down and indulge in all the worst hypotheticals that plague you.

3. **At the end of the half hour say, "See you tomorrow, worries."** Turn your attention to whatever activity is next (e.g., cooking, enjoying your kid/pet, working).

4. **Any time outside of the designated half hour, defer worries to the next mental litter box time.** Gently remind yourself that

right now is not the time to worry and that rest assured, you'll get to do it later/tomorrow.

Optional: During your mental litter box time, write down the worries that come up and sort them into two categories: "Can Control" versus "Cannot Control." For items in the "Can Control" column, write down what your next action step is (e.g., call to make an appointment today). For items in the "Cannot Control" column, let yourself worry about these as much as your mind wants to until the time is up. It may seem counterintuitive to worry on purpose, but the idea is to get the "Cannot Control" things out of your system during this designated worry time.

Tip: You can substitute "worry" with any type of thinking. You can use your mental litter box for rumination, self-doubt, self-recrimination, over-planning, regret, coming up with great comebacks that are too late to say, playing catchy songs on repeat—any mental process that is not helpful and not easy to shut off at night.

Sabotage #3: Lack of Adequate Wind Down Before Bedtime

If you're driving eighty miles per hour on the highway, you can't expect to be able to stop at the end of the exit ramp going that fast. You have to deliberately start slowing down well before the stop sign, or you'll drive right through it and into an intersection. Similarly, you have to start transitioning from get-it-done mode to let-it-go mode well before bedtime to help your body and mind wind down for sleep. If you are physically and mentally jazzed up and carrying that hyper-arousal into bed, you'll just be teaching your brain to have more conditioned arousal.

What to Do Instead

There are many ways to wind down, but when putting together your personal routine, consider following these principles:

Give Yourself a Clear Signal That the Get-It-Done Day Is Over

Perhaps closing your laptop with a satisfying thump at 8:00 P.M. is the signal, after which you do not even think about work or read the news. Maybe turning off the main house lights at 9:00 P.M. is the signal, leaving only your favorite lamp on for reading and your skincare routine. The signal could be at 10:00 P.M. when the chime on your phone signals you to wrap up whatever chore you're doing and change into pajamas, after which any to-do items will have to wait until tomorrow. If you do this consistently, your brain will learn to automatically begin the whole-body wind-down process at this signal.

Follow the Signal with a Roughly Consistent Ritual

Please don't get too precise or strict about this! We don't need a bedtime drill. It's simply helpful to have some consistency in the hour or so before bedtime, which will further condition your brain to automatically start a dearousal process. Perhaps you'll vary your activities from evening to evening, but always end it with a five-minute stretch and brushing your hair. Or you get your lunch ready for the next day and then cuddle with your partner. Maybe you always read before lights out, or pray.

During the Wind-Down Period, Do Activities That Are Inherently Pleasurable

If you're checking off anything on your regular to-do list, you're being too goal-oriented. Do something unproductive and nice for yourself, such as listening to music,* having a foot soak, snuggling with your cat, moisturizing your skin. Enjoy the moment with your five senses. You're switching from *doing* to *being*.

Don't Force It

This is the most important principle. Your wind-down routine is not meant to be a hammer that beats arousal down. It's merely your gentle invitation for sleepiness to come to you. Invitations are not always answered, and that's okay. Getting mad or trying to chase sleep down will only push it further away. If you're still not sleepy at the end of your bedtime routine, simply keep reading, stretching, watching TV, or doing something else enjoyable (outside of bed) until you feel sleepy.

Often, my patients wonder about exercise. You may have heard that exercising within a few hours of bedtime may be too stimulating and negatively affect sleep. Forget that. Unless you're doing an MMA fight right before bedtime, you're unlikely to be overly stimulating yourself. **In fact, exercise is beneficial for sleep, including increasing deep sleep.**† Besides, in our overly sedentary lives, I'd much rather you exercise whenever is convenient for you than worry about the timing.

Rules Are Meant to Be Broken

Sometimes a "perfect" bedtime routine is not possible and your own modifications are needed, which can actually be more helpful. For example, my routine goes something like this:

---

* Researchers have shown that listening to soothing music decreases the amount of time awake during the night. For once, something intuitive!

† Jan Stutz, Remo Eiholzer, and Christina M. Spengler, "Effects of Evening Exercise on Sleep in Healthy Participants: A Systematic Review and Meta-Analysis," *Sports Medicine* 49, no. 2 (2019): 269–87. https://doi.org/10.1007/S40279-018-1015-0.

7:30 P.M.: put toddler to bed, feel intense relief, collapse on the sofa like a sack of rocks

7:45 P.M.: do physical therapy exercises and chores with TV in the background

8:30 P.M. to 10:30 P.M.: write book/articles

10:30 P.M.: personal hygiene

10:45 P.M.: in bed with audiobook playing, lights out

You'll notice that two hours out of my three-and-a-quarter-hour evening is taken up by writing, which is very much a goal-oriented activity, and technically against my own "rule." But I love to write! I get antsy if I don't write, and end up going to bed with swirling ideas of what I wish I had written. I'm following the above principles in my own way: my "end of day" signal is putting my kid to bed, the consistent ritual that follows includes chores, writing, and personal hygiene, and my wind-down activities are almost always pleasurable.

The point is not to devise a "perfect" wind-down routine that strictly maximizes relaxation, but to enjoy your evening and tell your brain that all is safe and well.

DESIGN YOUR EVENING WIND-DOWN ROUTINE

1. The "doing" day is over at: _____ P.M. At this time, my signal to switch to "being" mode is _____ (e.g., gentle chime on my phone).
2. What I will include in my wind-down ritual after this signal:
   - ☐ Personal hygiene
   - ☐ Skincare or hair care routine
   - ☐ Drinking herbal tea

☐ Reading

☐ Chatting with my partner/kids/friends

☐ Cuddling my pets

☐ Laying out my clothes for tomorrow

☐ Listening to music

☐ Meditating

☐ Stretching

☐ Puttering

☐ Other: _____

☐ Other: _____

3. When I'm sleepy, I will go to bed, but I won't stay there if I be-come awake or feel myself putting effort into falling asleep.

Continuing Your Big Reset

You're familiar with this section by now. Let's see how you did with the Big Reset this week!

1. How Are Sleep Consolidation and Reversing Conditioned Arousal Going?

Assess your progress by looking at your Consensus Sleep Diary report (at www.ConsensusSleepDiary.com). Note these variables:

- **Sleep efficiency:** If you've been consistently following your sleep consolidation schedule and working on reversing conditioned arousal (i.e., only using the bed for sleep, and getting out of bed when you can't sleep) for more than two consecutive weeks, you should be in or close to the 85 to 95 percent range.
- **Total time in bed:** This should be very close to what you calcu-lated to be your time-in-bed window in chapter 6. If significantly

longer, that means you went to bed earlier than you were supposed to, or stayed in bed later than you were supposed to.

- **Time to fall asleep:** Generally, if this is under thirty minutes on average, or under thirty minutes on the vast majority of nights, you're falling asleep like a healthy sleeper. If not, you're likely still going to bed too early. Try staying up fifteen to thirty minutes later. Also, make sure you're keeping the same rise time every day!

- **Time awake in the middle of the night:** Ditto above. Continue getting out of bed during the night once you start to feel fully awake or have "racing mind."

- **Total sleep time:** This is the least important variable at this time. It could be longer, shorter, or the same as before—any of these cases wouldn't be meaningful. This is the last variable to change, and also the least stable and least meaningful for your healthy relationship with sleep. So, don't worry about this one right now.

2. Problem-Solve Hiccups with the Light + Movement Routine

Sometimes, despite our best intentions, it's difficult to implement the light + movement routine. Here are some common barriers:

- **You forget to do your scheduled activities, or it's hard to find time.** It's easy to let planned physical activity slip, especially if you're used to being sedentary or your environment isn't naturally set up for brightness. See if you can incentivize yourself by saving a treat (e.g., a favorite TV show, a dessert, or a bubble bath) for times when you *do* complete your planned activity. Better yet, get some social accountability by scheduling your activity (e.g., a walk) with a friend.

- **You don't feel motivated to do the activities.** Inertia is very real, especially if there is any depression simmering in the background. The key is not to wait until you feel motivated to do things—you may be waiting forever! You have to *do* things in order to feel better and to fan your motivation. You'll get on a positive spiral if you just brute force your way through the first few steps.

- **You can't get outside during the day.** It's okay if we need to tweak this. A light box at your workstation or kitchen counter, or better yet, light goggles that you can wear in the morning. Just twenty minutes in the morning goes a long way!

3. Update Your Time-in-Bed Window

Onward! Now you're in your fourth week of the Big Reset, and we'll tweak your time-in-bed window accordingly. Here's how.

- Note your past week's average sleep efficiency.
- **If it's above 90 percent, you get to have more time in bed this upcoming week.** Simply increase your previous time-in-bed window by fifteen minutes. This means you can either go to bed fifteen minutes earlier, or get up fifteen minutes later. Remember to maintain a consistent rise time throughout the week, with no more than an hour's "wiggle room."
- **If it's between 85 and 90 percent, let's hold steady with the schedule you've got from chapter 6 . . .** with the added permission to go to bed earlier than your scheduled time if you're very sleepy. That doesn't mean two hours earlier. More like give or take thirty minutes earlier, and only if you're sure you're sleepy.
- **If it's lower than 85 percent, see the problem-solving tips**

from chapters 5, 6, and above. You'll likely want to hold steady with the schedule you've got from chapter 6. If you've been consistently sticking with instructions, you should be seeing 85 percent-plus sleep efficiency by next week. This is the last week I'll ask you to "hang in there" before we let go of sleep consolidation and focus on other approaches.

What to Do This Upcoming Week

You're going to continue with the Big Reset, but now with four major components: (1) sleep consolidation, (2) reversing conditioned arousal, (3) continuing your light + movement routine, and (4) decreasing other arousal during the day. Altogether, your instructions include:

1. Get up at your regular rise time every day: _____ [insert new rise time].
2. Don't go to bed until your earliest allowed bedtime: _____ [insert new bedtime calculated above], or until you're sleepy.
3. Try not to nap or sleep in. *If your sleep efficiency was above 90 percent, OR if you have the occasional external demand that drastically shortens your sleep window (e.g., driving your spouse to the airport at 4:30 A.M.), you're now allowed a midday thirty-minute nap if sleepy.*
4. Don't do anything in bed other than sleeping. Sex and bedtime reading are allowed.
5. If you can't fall asleep (or can't fall back to sleep), get out of bed and do something for fun. Do not stay in bed or *try* to fall asleep.
6. Use your chapter 6 worksheets to continue your light + movement routine:

- Creating contrast between bright days and dim evenings
- Getting active (ideally outside) during the day at least three times per week

7. Use your chapter 7 worksheets to begin your daytime dearousal routine:
   - Mental litter box (or, if this is not helping, try walking or journaling)
   - Scheduled rest
   - Wind-down routine

BOTTOM LINE

- "Racing mind" is often the most frustrating thing about insomnia. You've already begun to quiet your racing mind by increasing your sleep drive and decreasing your conditioned arousal.
- To further let go of racing mind, make some changes during the day:
  » Give your brain a chance to process thoughts during the day.
  » Give yourself adequate daytime rest.
  » Give yourself a proper wind down before bedtime.
- This week, you will continue your Big Reset by recalculating your time-in-bed window based on last week's sleep log data. You will also continue to reverse conditioned arousal, engage in your light + movement routine, and use this chapter's worksheets (e.g., mental litter box) to help quiet your racing mind at night.
- Make sure to keep doing your sleep logs every day!

PART III

Going Deeper into the Relationship

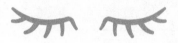

The Self-Fulfilling Prophecy

How Your Thoughts About Insomnia Feed Insomnia

K*ai often woke up during the night and had trouble getting back to sleep. He would lie there trying his best to relax, but he kept looking at the clock, counting down the hours he had left in the night, and thinking about just how terrible tomorrow was going to be. He would ask the darkness in desperation, "How am I going to function with this little sleep?" Eventually, he would drift back asleep and seemingly immediately be woken by the alarm. He would drag himself out of bed, thinking about how this insomnia thing is probably killing him. And it's putting a damper on everything, like going to the gym regularly, because now he doesn't feel like he can muster up the energy. He's feeling grumpy, resentful, and hopeless. And of course, he's tired.*

It's 3:00 A.M. You wake for no reason. Right away, you know you're not just vaguely aware of your surroundings . . . you're *really* awake. What's the first thought that comes to mind?

- "Oh no . . ."
- "Here we go again."

- "What's wrong with me?"
- "I won't be able to function tomorrow."
- "This sucks. I hate being awake during the night."
- "But I did everything right today! Why am I still waking up?"
- "Why do I have to deal with this? Nobody else has to deal with this."
- "If I can get myself to fall asleep within 15 minutes I will still have 3.75 hours to sleep, which means I will get a total of 2.75 + 3.75 = 6.5 hours total tonight, which is 18.75 percent less than I should get. This is bad because I'm already going on two nights in a row of getting only 6.75 hours per night, which means my sleep debt will be $(8 - 6.75) \times 2 + (8 - 6.5) \ldots$"

When you have a thought along those lines, how do you feel? Sometimes the thought is fleeting, and you can shrug it off easily. But if you're like most people I've worked with in the insomnia clinic, these thoughts often make you feel:

- Frustrated
- Anxious
- Resentful
- Angry
- Desperate
- Demoralized

Do any of these feelings help you to get back to sleep? Do any of them help you feel energized or happy the next day? Or do they spawn more irksome feelings and more spinning thoughts, so at best, you eventually drift back off into an irritable half sleep, and at worst, you're spiraling deeper into insomnia for the rest of the night? **This is the self-**

fulfilling prophecy of insomnia thoughts. In this cruel, Greek tragedy–style twist, the way we think about insomnia turns out to be one of the best fuels for keeping insomnia going.

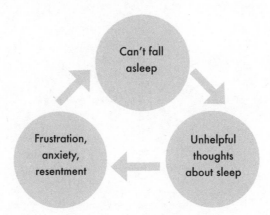

And this doesn't just apply to thoughts we have during the night. Have you ever had these thoughts during the day?

- "Insomnia is ruining my life."
- "Insomnia is slowly killing me."
- "I can't go on like this."
- "Sleep will never get better."
- "My body [or my brain, my sleep] has betrayed me."
- "Having kids [or insert other life event] ruined my sleep forever."
- "If it weren't for my sleep problems, I'd be able to _____"
  [insert highly desired activity].
- "I shouldn't schedule this trip [or party, project, etc.] because I won't be able to function well enough to enjoy it, given how bad my sleep is."

Do these thoughts make your relationship with sleep warm and fuzzy? Or do they turn up the pressure, fuel your frustration, stoke your anxiety, and add to the mental burden you carry from day to day? Most important, do these thoughts allow you to live your life more fully, or do they crowd your mental and emotional space with angst?

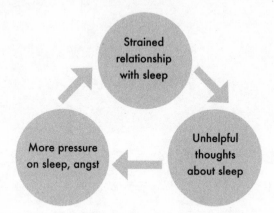

We keep coming back to hyperarousal, the main thing that insomnia feeds on 24/7. You've already worked hard to decrease your conditioned arousal, not-enough-rest arousal, circadian dysregulation arousal, and a few other types of arousal. Now it's time to look at another huge source of arousal—unhelpful thoughts about sleep.

We often underestimate just how much power our thoughts have. A single thought can change us from sleepy to alert, and a habit of thinking can change sleep from a friend to an adversary. After all, why would sleep want to spend time with us if we keep putting pressure on it to perform, blame it for our problems, and always expect the worst from it? If we want to be friends with sleep and for it to accept our nighttime invitation, we need to reexamine the way we think about sleep and insomnia.

This is what Kai and I spent most of our time working on. He had a tendency, in his own words, to "think up a storm." In the past, when he tried to "turn off his brain," or turn his negative thoughts about sleep into positive ones, he found himself spinning in mental circles and getting even more frustrated. Sometimes, he'd suddenly realize he had been ruminating about insomnia for his whole morning commute, and was even more vexed than when he woke up. But once he realized that his automatic thoughts about sleep were leading him down an unhelpful path, he began to respond more intentionally to them.* With practice, developing a more helpful perspective became second nature. Kai said that people around him even commented on how much more relaxed he seemed! If you can do what Kai did and approach your thoughts with more flexibility, you'll be going a long way to healing your relationship with sleep. Let's get started.

Step 1: Become Aware of Your Automatic Thoughts About Sleep

The first step to changing anything is to understand it. This is how automatic thoughts usually work:

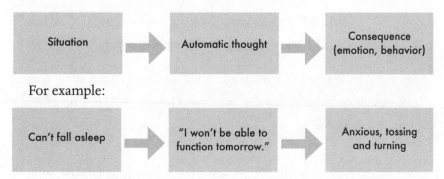

For example:

See how the automatic thought ("I won't be able to function tomorrow") is the bridge between the situation (can't fall asleep) and the emotional and behavioral consequences (feeling anxious and struggling in bed)? The reason we call these thoughts "automatic" is because they can happen so quickly and under-the-radar that we're often not even aware we've had them. We may experience a seemingly direct link from

---

* Allison G. Harvey, Ann L. Sharpley, Melissa J. Ree, Katheen Stinson, and David M. Clark, "An Open Trial of Cognitive Therapy for Chronic Insomnia," *Behaviour Research and Therapy* 45, no. 10 (2007): 2491–2501. https://doi.org/10.1016/J.BRAT.2007.04.007.

not being able to fall asleep to feeling terrible, as if being awake at night inevitably results in feeling this way. I can already hear you protesting, "But of course being awake at night feels terrible!" Historically, this has been your experience. But what if being awake doesn't *have to* mean anxiety and struggle? What if it went something like this:

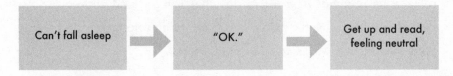

Can't fall asleep → "OK." → Get up and read, feeling neutral

Believe it or not, this whole process is more within your control than you think, though it will take practice. There's no need to rush. To get there, let's start with noticing our automatic thoughts about sleep.* To do so, use the thought record on page 165 for a week.

What If I'm Having Trouble Identifying My Automatic Thoughts?

Automatic thoughts are very hard to catch! Don't worry if it doesn't come naturally—you're not the only one. Here are two tips for noticing automatic thoughts:

1. Work backward. If you find yourself feeling frustrated, anxious, or resentful about your sleep, note them in the third column and ask, "Why am I feeling this way? What was I just thinking? What *about* this situation is making me feel so bad?" Even if the answer you come up with seems really obvious (e.g., "I'm not getting enough sleep"), write it down.

---

* And let's do it without any judgment, because we don't need guilt and self-recrimination in the mix too! If you catch yourself thinking, "I *shouldn't* be thinking like this" or "This is a stupid thought," remind yourself that thoughts are just your brain's way of trying to help. Berating yourself adds to the anxiety/ frustration soup. The best way to teach your brain what's helpful versus what's not is to keep giving it gentle feedback (e.g., "This is an interesting thought. Let's see if it's helpful for the current situation.")

SITUATION	AUTOMATIC THOUGHT	CONSEQUENCES (EMOTIONS, BEHAVIORS)
Can't fall asleep. It's been at least an hour.	"I won't be able to function tomorrow."	Frustrated, desperate Trying hard to relax

2. Keep asking, "So what?" If you identify a thought but it doesn't seem inherently unhelpful (e.g., "It's 4:00 A.M." or "I'm awake again"), ask yourself, "So what if it's 4:00 A.M.? So what if I'm awake again?" You'll find that the *true* automatic thought causing the angst is there. Perhaps, "This means I only have two more hours of possible sleep left, and that's not enough. I won't be able to function tomorrow."

What if My Automatic Thoughts Are Already Accurate or Positive?

No problem! We're not trying to judge the thoughts. It doesn't matter if they're true or false, positive or negative. We're just trying to understand how you think about sleep, and what these thoughts lead to. Chances are, you'll have a mix of differently flavored thoughts about sleep.

What if My Automatic Thoughts Are Really Vague?

Sometimes, all people can articulate is, "Oh no" or "Here we go again." But try to go further, because we need more substance to work with here. What specifically is making you go, "Oh no"? Here we go again with what? Perhaps it's, "Oh no, now I'm going to be awake for hours," or, "Here we go with the battle to fall asleep again . . . it's going to take so much effort."

What if All My Automatic Thoughts Are in the Form of Questions?

Often, thought records are full of questions like, "Why is this happening to me?" and "Why am I not sleeping?" and "How am I going to function tomorrow?" It's very important to nail down the statements behind these questions, because when we start working to dissect these thoughts, we'll need statements to work with. So try to answer the questions you pose. For example, what you're really thinking may be, "It's not fair that this is happening to me," "I can't predict or control my sleep," or "I'm not going to function tomorrow."

Step 2: Examine Your Automatic Thoughts About Sleep

Remember, there's no need to rush. Take your time with Step 1 and make sure you have at least a few automatic thoughts noted, and you feel like you've got the hang of identifying them as they come up. This first step may very well take a whole week, and that's okay. When you're ready, it's time to start examining these thoughts. When you're first practicing this skill, you may want to wait until the daytime, when you can think more clearly and not risk overanalyzing while in the middle of a frustrating insomnia bout at 2:00 A.M. As this skill becomes easier to do, you can start using it in the moment, whenever an unhelpful automatic thought pops up. For now, choose one example from your thought record and ask yourself: Is this thought helpful? If the answer is "Yes," that's great! That means whatever the thought is, it's making you feel good and helping your sleep. If not, ask yourself some more questions:

1. **Is this thought based in fact or in fear? Is it consistent with the scientific facts about sleep we've learned in this book?**

Sometimes, what you've previously heard about sleep will sneak into your mind again and say, "I'm going to get dementia if I don't get eight hours of sleep per night," or "I'm sleep deprived." I invite you to leaf through chapters 1 and 2 again to refresh on facts about sleep and insomnia. You may find that a more accurate response to your thought might be, "I may not need eight hours of sleep" or "I have insomnia, not sleep deprivation. The scary consequences of sleep deprivation don't apply to me."

2. **If this thought is a prediction, have there been times when this wasn't true? Are there counterexamples to my prediction?**

For example, "I'm going to be useless tomorrow." Have there been times when you didn't sleep much but functioned the next day anyway? Conversely, have there been times when you slept a lot but still had a crummy day? Are there other things that contribute to your having a good or bad day? If so, what does this mean about how much tomorrow hinges on your sleep tonight?

3. **If my prediction does come true, what's the worst that will come of it? How likely is that outcome? Will I be able to cope?**

For example, "I'm going to be so tired tomorrow." Perhaps the worst possible scenario is that you function so terribly that you make a catastrophic mistake at work and get fired. How often has this happened in the past, on the many occasions when you've had bad nights? Is it likely that it will happen tomorrow? What steps would you take to remedy the situation or cope with the fallout?

4. **Am I putting too much pressure on my sleep? Am I unfairly blaming sleep or expecting too much?**

For example, "My body has betrayed me. I should be able to sleep like I used to." Whenever "should" sneaks into one of your automatic thoughts about sleep, there's a good chance you're putting too much pressure on sleep. Whenever you're talking about your sleep as if it owes you, you're likely being unfair.

5. **What's a more fair, balanced, and accurate way to think about this situation?**

Notice that I didn't say to come up with a more positive thought. Simply putting on rose-colored glasses doesn't tend to work well, because we know when we're fooling ourselves. Instead, we want to be realistic and fair. Sometimes we can do this simply by completing the sentence. For example, "I've had insomnia for so long . . ." can become, "I've had insomnia for so long . . . it sucks! But now I'm rebuilding a good relationship with sleep. I can see hope."

MY POCKET SOCRATES

Socrates was famous for teaching through asking questions. Using his approach can help you better understand your automatic thoughts about sleep. Feel free to copy these questions onto a flash card to carry around or put on your night table, so you can always consult your pocket Socrates:

- Is this thought based in fact or in fear?
- If this thought is a prediction, have there been times when it wasn't true?
- If my prediction does come true, what's the worst that will come of it? Would I be able to cope?
- Am I putting too much pressure on my sleep, or being unfair?
- What's a more fair, balanced, and accurate way to think about this situation?

Step 3: Practice Shifting to a More Helpful Perspective

When you examined your automatic thoughts, you already began to practice approaching sleep with a more helpful attitude. Let's see Kai in action to see how we can further practice. First, he and I noticed his automatic thoughts about sleep and identified three frequent ones, then we imagined putting on ancient Greek robes and role-played Socrates talking with one of his students:

Automatic Thought #1: "If I Don't Fall Asleep Very Soon, I Won't Be Able to Function Tomorrow."

Kai: If I don't fall asleep very soon, I won't be able to function tomorrow.

Socrates: Have you had bad nights before, similar to this one?

Kai: Yes, I've had insomnia for years. I'm often awake for at least an hour, sometimes two or three, during the night.

Socrates: Have you ever been able to function the next day, after one of these bad nights?

Kai: I guess so. I always seem to push through.

Socrates: Is it possible that you'll be able to pull that off again tomorrow?

Kai: Yes, I'll probably pull through. I just make mistakes or forget things if I don't sleep enough.

Socrates: Have you made mistakes or forgotten things even after a good night of sleep?

Kai: Yes, I guess I have.

Socrates: So, does your functioning entirely depend on how much you sleep?

Kai: No, it depends on a lot of other things too, like whether I eat breakfast and how busy things are at work.

Socrates: What is the worst thing that will happen if you *do* make a mistake or forget something?

Kai: I'll apologize and correct the mistake. Unless it's catastrophic, then I might lose my job.

Socrates: How often have you made mistakes catastrophic enough to cost you your job?

Kai: Never.

Socrates: What might be a more accurate and fair version of your initial prediction that you won't be able to function if you don't fall asleep soon?

Kai: I may feel tired and not be my best self tomorrow, but I'll probably still be able to function well. And if I'm not perfect, that's okay. It won't be the end of the world.

How do you think Kai feels before versus after having this conversation with Socrates? Which version of Kai will sleep better for the rest of tonight, and for the nights to come?

Automatic Thought #2: "Insomnia Is Slowly Killing Me."

Kai: Insomnia is slowly killing me.

Socrates: Hi! Me again. How do you know insomnia is killing you?

Kai: I've read that sleep deprivation is bad for your heart, brain, gut, and everything else.

Socrates: Is insomnia the same thing as sleep deprivation, based on what you've learned from *Hello Sleep*?

Kai: No. Sleep deprivation is when external things (like night-shift work) prevent me from sleeping. Insomnia is when I have enough opportunity to sleep but my own brain doesn't let me.

Socrates: Would you say, then, that your belief is based in fact or in fear?

Kai: I guess I'm just afraid that insomnia is killing me. So it's based in fear.

Socrates: And is this thought that insomnia is killing you helpful for you at this moment?

Kai: No, it just makes me more anxious.

Socrates: What's a possible helpful response to this thought?

Kai: I don't know for a fact that insomnia is killing me. I don't like it, but it's probably not causing harm the way that sleep deprivation would. In any case, I'm working on improving my sleep so I'm going in a good direction.

Which version of Kai, before versus after this conversation with Socrates, has a better relationship with sleep? Which one is increasing versus decreasing arousal?

Automatic Thought #3: "If It Weren't for My Sleep Problems, I'd Be Able to Regularly Go to the Gym."

Kai: If it weren't for my sleep problems, I'd be able to regularly go to the gym.

Socrates: What specifically is stopping you from going to the gym today?

Kai: I can't go because I'm so tired, because I didn't sleep well.

Socrates: Are there any other possible reasons for feeling tired?

Kai: I guess I might be stressed out and in a crummy mood. My teenager seems especially unreasonable today.

Socrates: Is it fair to blame your tiredness and gym hiatus entirely on sleep problems?

Kai: Maybe sometimes it's just an excuse. I just feel so blah and unmotivated.

Socrates: Is there any chance that going to the gym could improve your mood or make you feel more energized?

Kai: Yes, that's why I used to love going to the gym. I wish I could still go regularly.

Socrates: Have you tried going to the gym recently even after not sleeping well?

Kai: No, I haven't gone in a long time.

Socrates: Do you know for a fact that you *can't* go? What could be the worst outcome?

Kai: I guess I could try. Worst case is that I'll only do part of my regular workout, feel exhausted, and come home.

Which version of Kai is more likely to go to the gym and reap the benefits of exercise today? Which one is going to have more sleep drive, better mood, and less stress? Channel your inner Socrates and try this for yourself! You can use an expanded version of the thought record to keep track:

SITUATION	AUTOMATIC THOUGHT	CONSEQUENCES (EMOTIONS, BEHAVIORS)	MORE ACCURATE, FAIR, OR HELPFUL THOUGHT	CONSEQUENCES (EMOTIONS, BEHAVIORS)
Woke up at night and partner is just snoring away.	I'm the only one in the family with insomnia, even though I have better sleep hygiene than everyone. This is so unfair.	Frustrated. Resentful. Felt like partner's snoring got even louder.	I don't like that I'm so lonely in my insomnia experience, but it's nobody's fault. And I'm proud of myself for working on restoring a good relationship with sleep.	Felt slightly better. Got up and listened to a podcast I enjoyed.

Remember that the ultimate goal here isn't to take your thoughts to court. We're not here to win an argument against our brain! **Focus less on what's true versus false (this dichotomy doesn't always make sense anyway), and more on what's helpful versus unhelpful.** We can hold on to the idea that, yes, it sucks that you have insomnia while nobody else in your family even understands what you're going through. It *is* unfair. But is it helpful to keep hammering on this thought in the middle of the night? Perhaps it's more helpful to get up and enjoy a little extra "me" time with your favorite podcast.

Be patient with yourself. Approaching your unhelpful thoughts like Socrates is a skill, and it needs practice just like riding a bike. Try to catch at least one automatic thought per day and spend a couple of minutes going through your pocket Socrates questions to see what other perspectives you gain. If you don't have sleep-related automatic thoughts that often, congratulations! Still try to practice noticing and examining unhelpful thoughts about other things, such as your anxiety about an upcoming work deadline, or worries about your child not eating broccoli. This tool can be applied to any situation.

What to Do This Upcoming Week

At this point, if you've been doing the Big Reset for about four weeks, you should be seeing changes in your sleep log data, including sleep efficiencies mostly above 85 percent (and averaging above 85 percent over the week), shorter time to fall asleep on average (if you started out with taking thirty-plus minutes to fall asleep), shorter time awake during the night on average (if you started out with thirty-plus minutes awake), and less frequent bouts of long wakefulness during the night. Hopefully, you're also feeling more confident and satisfied with your sleep.

If the above sounds like your progress—congratulations! Great work. At this point, you don't have to be as strict about things as during the Big Reset. For example:

- You can go to bed earlier than your previously prescribed bedtime if you're truly sleepy.
- You can give yourself a little more wiggle room on when to get up, but still keep your rise time to within one hour.
- You can take a short midday nap (less than thirty minutes) just for fun, if you feel sleepy and would enjoy it.
- Still get out of bed if you feel wide awake and can't fall asleep,

whether it's the beginning or middle of the night. But if you're feeling cozy and content, and may be drifting in and out of sleep, feel free to stay put.

We're moving toward our ultimate goal—not having to be so regimented about sleep or treat it as a project. **Now that we've successfully used the Big Reset to increase sleep drive and decrease conditioned arousal, you and sleep have a clean slate for rebuilding your relationship. You can now turn your focus to the more nuanced and emotional aspects of this relationship, part of which is to listen to your body and trust what it's telling you.**

But the Big Reset Isn't Working. What's Going On?

If you're not seeing the changes I described above, there are a few possibilities why:

- You might need to hang in there for one more week. Sometimes, people seem to not progress for a few weeks, but suddenly it clicks. Try keeping with the Big Reset for one more week if you think this might be the case, after which you can say you've given it your best shot, let it go, and turn your attention to the skills in part III.
- Your insomnia-perpetuating factors are more about the way you think about sleep, and not so much about the way you act around sleep. You'll notice that part II (The Big Reset) is mostly about what to *do* differently, and part III (Going Deeper into the Relationship) is more about how to *think* differently. Try out the skills in part III and see if these resonate more.
- Your body needs more time to benefit from the light + movement routine, or the daytime rest plan, which you've only re-

cently started implementing, or it needs a bigger dose of these changes. Our bodies and brains don't always respond overnight to helpful things we do. Let's keep working on making these investments!

- You might have big sources of arousal that we haven't covered yet, such as excessive caffeine, history of trauma, ongoing severe stress, or a bed partner that severely disturbs your sleep. These might be so significant that decreases in other forms of arousal are overshadowed. Feel free to browse other chapters in part III and part IV that seem relevant to your situation. It's less important to go in sequence from here onward.

- You may also have another sleep or circadian rhythm disorder, or a medical condition (or medication) that significantly disrupts your sleep and makes it hard for insomnia therapy to fully work. It's always worth checking with your doctor about this possibility, including reviewing your medications and walking through potential red flags for disorders like obstructive sleep apnea or periodic limb movement disorder (see chapter 16).

In any case, it never hurts to do your light + movement routine and to protect your rest time during the day. Hopefully, these are becoming easier to incorporate into your daily life. All together, your instructions for this week include:

1. Get up at your regular rise time every day: _____.
2. Don't go to bed until you're sleepy.
3. Keep the bed for sleeping only. (Sex and reading are still allowed!)
4. If you feel wide awake or frustrated, get out of bed. Don't try to force sleep.

5. Keep prioritizing light, movement, and rest.
6. Use chapter 8 worksheets (pages 165 and 173) to notice and examine your automatic thoughts about sleep. Practice shifting your perspective to a more fair, accurate, or helpful one.

BOTTOM LINE

- The way we think about sleep has a powerful effect on our relationship with it.
- Often, our unhelpful automatic thoughts about insomnia can make it harder to sleep in the moment, keeping insomnia around long term.
- To get out of this self-fulfilling prophecy, we can take three steps:
  » Become aware of our automatic thoughts about sleep and their consequences.
  » Examine these thoughts using your pocket Socrates questions.
  » Practice approaching sleep-related situations with more fair, accurate, and helpful perspectives.
- If the Big Reset has improved your sleep log numbers, great! You can be less strict with your bedtime and shift more toward listening to your body for sleepiness cues.
- Keep doing your sleep logs!

Just Sleep, Dammit!

*Why Insomnia Thrives on Sleep Effort and
How to Let It Go*

How much time would you like to dedicate to working on sleep in the next week? Next year? Rest of your life? What percent of your days and nights would you like to spend on the sleep project? If you live to the venerable age of ninety-nine, you will have spent twenty-five to thirty-three years either sleeping or trying to sleep. How many of those years would you like to spend managing, coaxing, or strategizing sleep, and how much overtime work are you willing to put in?

If you're struggling to come up with an answer to these questions, perhaps it's because you haven't considered the most obvious one: none. Perhaps you haven't dared to consider that this is even possible—to not spend any time *working* on sleep. After all, if it was that easy, you wouldn't be reading this book. But suspend your disbelief and fantasize with me for a moment. What if

- you don't have to know what time it is right now, during the night, and don't have to calculate just how much time you have left to sleep?

- you don't have to review just how bad your sleep has been lately, counting the hours of "sleep debt" you must be accumulating?
- you don't have to fall back to sleep right now, at 3:38 A.M., even though you have a big presentation to give tomorrow?
- you don't have to even consider how much sleep you'll get when someone invites you to a camping vacation?
- you don't have to figure out why your partner falls asleep as soon as they hit the pillow, even though your sleep hygiene is better than theirs?
- you don't have to silently scream, "Just sleep, dammit!" into the darkness . . . ever again?

You may think, "Well, of course, all this would be fabulous. As soon as I'm sleeping well, it will no longer be such hard work." **But what if it's the other way around?** What if you can let go of *sleep effort* right now, and as a result, enjoy better sleep?

What Is Sleep Effort?

Sleep effort involves anything you intentionally do or think in an attempt to induce sleep, or to become a better sleeper.* See if these are familiar:

- Researching the best pillow or mattress for sleep
- Trying really hard to clear your mind or turn off your brain at night
- Trying to figure out the best sleep position or perfect bedtime routine
- Making sure you go to bed early so you have plenty of time to get enough hours

* Niall M. Broomfield and Colin A. Espie, "Towards a Valid, Reliable Measure of Sleep Effort," *Journal of Sleep Research* 14, no. 4 (2005): 401–7. https://doi.org/10.1111/J.1365-2869.2005.00481.X.

- Asking your family to be extra quiet after you go to bed at night or before you get up in the morning
- Checking the time when you wake up during the night
- Strategizing about your sleep medication (Should I take a full versus half dose tonight?)
- Trying to drum up a positive attitude about sleep leading up to bedtime
- Avoiding drinking liquids in the late evening to minimize nighttime urination
- Using special sleep meditations, soundtracks, or "binaural beats" to try to induce sleep
- Buying products that are supposedly sleep inducing (e.g., lavender mist)
- Going down an internet "research" rabbit hole about sleep and insomnia

We care about sleep effort because it's one of the biggest perpetuating factors for chronic insomnia. After all, how can we expect to have a good relationship with sleep if it's all work and no fun? Sleep effort is a particularly slippery problem because it's so counterintuitive. Everything else in your life improves when you work harder at it, doesn't it? You have to be intentional and disciplined about your exercise regimen if you're training for a triathlon. You have to study and practice if you want to learn Spanish. We've all been taught that hard work is a virtue.

But when it comes to sleep, hard work often backfires. For Denise, a particularly diligent woman I worked with, sleep had become a part-time job. She was constantly thinking about how much she had (or hadn't) slept, strategizing about how to get more sleep, and trying every method she could find on the internet to perfect her sleep habits. She became convinced at one point that meditation would be the answer to her sleep problems. But when she went all-in on meditation—attending a weekend meditation retreat, buying meditation apps, researching the best sleep meditation music, etc.—she found herself even more frustrated at night. Sometimes meditating seemed to work, giving her a glimpse of hope, but often, the harder she meditated, the further sleep seemed to slip away. During the night, when she woke up, she couldn't help checking the clock. When asked why she did this, Denise said, "Well, just to know what time it is."

Being "bad at falling asleep" became even more entrenched into her identity as a person, so she started turning down social opportunities. For example, when her friends invited her over for Saturday evening drinks, she stayed home because she didn't want to be out too late and set herself up for even less sleep (she calculated that if it usually took her one and a half hours to fall asleep, she'd better be in bed by 9:30 P.M. and hope for falling asleep at 11:00 P.M.). Being at home by herself just made her bored and miserable because she was missing out on the fun.

Between researching, strategizing, working hard at meditating, and prioritizing protecting sleep, Denise was putting a lot of effort into this engineering problem. What did all of her sleep effort behaviors have in common? *They resulted in hyperarousal.* They either made her more anxious about sleep, drew more attention to her fears about sleep, or increased the frustration she had about her sleep. By now, we know that hyperarousal is insomnia's strongest fuel, and Denise didn't realize that she herself was pouring it on the fire.

How to Let Go of Sleep Effort

If you grew up watching cartoons, you are familiar with quicksand.* If you find yourself knee-deep in it and sinking, what's the worst thing

---

* As a kid growing up in China and watching American cartoons, I really thought the United States was full of quicksand pits based on their frequent depiction. I'm disappointed in never having encountered one in all my years living here as an adult.

you can do? That's right—struggle. What should you do instead? That's right—stop moving and lay flat.

Dealing with insomnia is quite similar. If you find yourself stuck in a bout of wakefulness at night, the worst thing you can do is struggle—rail against the injustice of it all, try hard to relax (dammit), think about how you *should* be sleeping, etc. This struggle will only sink you deeper into insomnia by firing up your fight-or-flight system and feeding your conditioned arousal.

This "stop the struggle" idea (and the quicksand metaphor) is borrowed from Acceptance and Commitment Therapy,* an evidence-based psychotherapy approach developed by psychologist Dr. Steven Hayes, a professor at the University of Nevada, and popularized by writers like Dr. Russ Harris (*The Happiness Trap: Stop Struggling, Start Living*).† The core of this approach rests on psychological flexibility, which I think is key when it comes to sleep effort. Instead of struggling the same way you always have against being awake at night, can we be flexible and respond in other, perhaps counterintuitive, ways? Let's get back to the original quicksand metaphor: What's the sleep equivalent of "stop moving and lay flat"? Here are some concrete ways to stop the struggle.

Stop the Struggle Tip #1: Accept Reality (and Say It Out Loud)

Notice how the lay-flat response to quicksand works *with* reality, instead of *against* it? You're acknowledging that, yes, you're in quicksand, it's already happening, and quicksand won't magically become not-quicksand

---

* Steven C. Hayes, "Acceptance and Commitment Therapy, Relational Frame Theory, and the Third Wave of Behavioral and Cognitive Therapies," *Behavior Therapy* 35, no. 4 (2004): 639–65. https://doi.org/10.1016/S0005-7894(04)80013-3.

† Russ Harris, *The Happiness Trap: How to Stop Struggling and Start Living* (Wollombi, Australia: Exisle Publishing Limited, 2008), 246. https://books.google.com/books/about/The_Happiness_Trap.html?id=K9m-EI04pgcC.

just because you and your flailing limbs really, really want this reality to change. When you're wide awake at night, you can similarly acknowledge that, yes, you're awake right now, it's already happening, and your wakefulness won't magically become sleepiness just because you and your flailing brain really, really want this reality to change.

In other words, you can choose to accept reality. That means to notice what is happening in the moment without analyzing, evaluating, or striving. It is simply to acknowledge that what is, is. Here's what the difference between accepting and not accepting reality looked like for Denise:

STRUGGLING AGAINST REALITY	ACCEPTING REALITY
Really, brain? Right now you're just going to be awake for no reason?	I'm awake.
Come *on*, just relax, dammit!	My body is not sleepy right now.
I did everything right. There's no reason why I should be awake right now.	I see a pattern of lights across the ceiling.
This is so unfair. It's torture.	I hear the air conditioning's hum.
Just clear your mind. Clear your mind. Clear your mind.	I feel the sheets against my skin.
Why isn't this relaxation exercise working??	I notice thoughts going through my head.
I'm going to be so mad if I don't fall back to sleep within . . .	
Why is it 3:47 A.M.?	
Life would be so much easier if I could just sleep well.	
I can't keep going like this.	

In my professional and personal experience, people rarely win fights against reality. We all know this, but it sometimes doesn't stop us from trying, and switching gears from struggling to accepting is not easy to do! But simply asking yourself, "Am I flailing in quicksand right now?" might just be the reminder you need to take a pause and say (out loud), "I guess I'm not sleepy. Okay." And that's a very good start.

Stop the Struggle Tip #2: What Would a Good Sleeper Do?

When you feel sleep effort creeping up on you, say, in the form of a pestering doubt about travel plans you made ("Is getting to the hotel this late going to mess up my sleep for that night?"), pause and ask yourself, **"What would I do in this situation if I didn't have insomnia in my life?"** Usually, the answer is, "I wouldn't worry about sleep, or even take it into account."

It helps to have a role model in mind—someone you consider an effortlessly great sleeper. Then you can ask yourself, "What would so-and-so do in this situation?" When Denise did this thought experiment, I could almost see a light bulb turn on over her head. She said, "My sister Claire is the best sleeper in the world. I hate her. And if she were in my shoes, she would just go to her friend's house and enjoy a cocktail and gossip and not even think about sleep. Because what's the worst that could happen if she went to bed late?"

What about meditation? Denise thought about it and said, "Claire would go, 'Screw meditating. It's stressing me out.' And she would get up and do some laundry or watch TV instead."

We decided on a mantra for Denise: WWCD—What Would Claire Do? This was a game changer. Denise started acting as if she didn't have a big insomnia shadow hanging over her all the time, and instead, lived her life the way she wanted to. Then, one week later, she realized that she hadn't thought about sleep for at least three days in a row. How liberating!

Denise benefited from the fact that our bodies take hints from our actions. If our actions indicate that sleep is fragile, our bodies will make us more vigilant about wakefulness at night, making us more prone to waking up and staying awake. If our actions indicate that changes to our sleep routine are dangerous, our bodies will react with anxiety whenever our sleep routine is disrupted. However, if our actions indicate that sleep is resilient and adaptable, and that our relationship with sleep is solid enough to withstand some turbulence, our bodies will tone down the arousal, resting assured that it doesn't need to be on guard for danger.

Stop the Struggle Tip #3: Get Out of Your Head and into Your Body

If I could get a tattoo of any line from this book it would be, "Get out of your head and into your body."

Our minds are wonderful—they are what allowed the human species to be so successful. But sometimes they overdo things to the point of being counterproductive. For example, sometimes our minds project a chain of what-ifs far down the line, making our bodies borrow stress from a hypothetical future of worst-case scenarios. Or our minds read too much into coincidences and try to recreate that time we had great sleep by taking the exact same dose of trazodone at the exact hour with our feet pointing in the exact direction, only to shine a spotlight on the (false) idea that our sleep is fragile, making our bodies more nervous as we get close to bedtime.

Our bodies, on the other hand, are simpler creatures. They're great at gathering data from the real world of the here and now, keeping us grounded to what's really happening and how threatening a situation really is (or isn't). When we ask our bodies for a status update, we'll get a straightforward answer, usually with less melodrama than the mind would produce.

Of course, sometimes our bodies do not seem like welcoming places to be. They might be seized with pain or burning with anxiety, and for many of us, this may even be a chronic state if we have experienced trauma or have a disorder like fibromyalgia. This can, understandably, make us want to be anywhere *but* in the body. **Yet, even in these cases, we actually experience less pain and anxiety when we accept and allow those bodily sensations, instead of struggling against them in our minds.*** It's always easier to go *with* reality than against it.

If you're familiar with the increasingly popular concept of mindfulness, you may recognize that "get out of your head and into your body" is really the same idea. Mindfulness originated in Eastern philosophy, and it means being aware of the present moment without judgment. This concept got entangled with that of meditation, an umbrella term for a diverse range of consciousness-changing techniques, and now there's often a misconception that mindfulness is about slowing down your breath, clearing your mind, or repeating a soothing mantra. In fact, it's in some ways the opposite of these popular meditation concepts—it's all about *letting go* of control, refraining from imposing your judgment or will on your body and environment, and observing what's going on instead of manipulating it. Often, when I bring up mindfulness, patients (Denise included) are skeptical because they've already tried breathing techniques or had gone to meditation class, and what they learned was either not feasible to do regularly, not helpful, or can even be actively frustrating.[†] But once they learn the true meaning of mindfulness and start practicing the acceptance that comes with it, it becomes a paradigm-shifting idea that helps with sleep and everything else in life.

There are other books that go into much more depth about mindfulness (see the appendix for recommended resources), but for now, let's dip our toe in with some accessible "get out of your head and into your body" practices.

---

* Lara Hilton, Susanne Hempel, Brett A. Ewing, Eric Apaydin, Lea Xenakis, Sydne Newberry, Ben Colaiaco, et al., "Mindfulness Meditation for Chronic Pain: Systematic Review and Meta-Analysis," *Annals of Behavioral Medicine* 51, no. 2 (2017): 199–213. https://doi.org/10.1007/S12160-016-9844-2.

† Please know that I am not trying to discourage meditation. This is beneficial for many people, and there is nothing wrong with meditating if you like it. In fact, one way to practice mindfulness is through mindfulness-based meditations. I just want to clarify that if you've tried some forms of meditation and didn't like them, that doesn't mean mindfulness is not for you.

THE 5-4-3-2-1 EXERCISE

This mindfulness exercise can be done anywhere, anytime. It's particularly helpful when you feel yourself getting into a rumination spiral. Simply pause and ask yourself,

- What are 5 things I see around me?
- What are 4 things I hear?
- What are 3 things I can feel with my body?
- What are 2 things I can smell?
- What is 1 thing I can taste? (Replace with another thing you feel with your body, or an emotion, if you don't have anything to taste.)

When I do this exercise for the first time with patients, they tend to do two nonmindful things:

1. **Rushing through the checklist:** Slow down! It's not a competition to get this done as quickly as possible. Our brains are so good at naming objects that we barely have to pay attention to say, "phone, picture, cup, trash can, pen." But the point isn't just to name objects, it's to really *see* them. Observe visual qualities or previously unnoticed details instead, like, "There's a smudge of dust on my phone's touchscreen, the picture is a little faded in one corner, the sunlight is gleaming on the lip of this cup, the trash can has a sticker on it that I never noticed, and the pen is royal blue in this light."

2. **Analyzing or judging what they're experiencing:** Often, little judgments sneak through like, "I feel this itch on my ear that's been there all day . . . a mosquito must have snuck inside" or "I can smell the stale socks from my son's room, it's gross" or "I see the

flowers on my desk . . . I love those." This is how we get into our heads, away from our bodies. Instead, allow yourself to simply notice, period. No interpretation or analysis needed. Allow yourself to simply *be* with the sensation you sense, wide open with curiosity as if you were a newborn baby.

When you really do the 5–4–3–2–1 exercise, you're simply experiencing the here and now through your five senses. And you're so focused on the here and now that you're not borrowing stress from the future or spinning yarns in your mind.

THE MINDFUL BREATH

You can do this one anytime, anywhere, too, since your breath is always with you. No need to barricade yourself in a quiet room or find a soothing bamboo forest. Wherever you are, simply breathe.

- Notice what your breath feels like. How does the air entering your nose feel? How does it feel as it leaves your nose or mouth? How does your body move as you breathe?
- Don't change anything about your breath, or judge it as good or bad.
- Don't fight it when you notice other thoughts drifting in (e.g., "Am I picking up milk from the store, or just eggs?" "Is this mindfulness thing even helpful?"). It's okay to have thoughts.
- Notice these thoughts swirling in your head, gently set them off to the side, and turn your attention back to the breath when you're ready.
- Keep noticing the sensations of your breath.

I highly recommend trying this one with guided audio, which you can find for free on the internet. See the appendix for recommended ones.

THE BODY SCAN

This is my favorite. As a person with chronic back pain, the body scan has been a total game changer for how I relate to my body and pain. It's also simple and doable anywhere, anytime:

- Start with a mindful breath to get into the here and now.
- Bring your attention to the little toe on your left foot. What does it feel? Wiggle it to get in touch with any sensations there. No need to judge anything as good or bad; we're just here to notice.
- Bring your attention to the rest of your toes. What do they feel?
- Bring your attention to the soles and backs of your feet. What do they feel?
- How about your ankles? Shins? Calves?
- Taking your time, slowly walk your attention through each part of your body, noticing sensations without offering any judgment, interpretation, command, or attempt to avoid them.
- Even if there are unpleasant sensations like pain, we're just here to experience it. Allow yourself to linger there. Ask what form the pain takes. What color is it if it had a color? Does it wax and wane, or is it steady? Be curious.

Remember that the point is not necessarily to make your body feel better or more relaxed. We're simply trying to get in touch with it. This teaches us to be more aware of the body's needs, such as becoming more familiar with what it feels like to be sleepy (versus tired). It also teaches us to listen to and trust our bodies, instead of imposing arbitrary expectations. In other words, we're experiencing more being, less struggling.

Stop the Struggle Bonus Tip: Cover Up Your Clock

There is no reason for you to know what time it is when you're not falling asleep or when you wake up during the night. If you've already set your morning alarm, you don't need to keep track of the time to avoid being late. If you're following the general guideline of "getting out of bed when you feel very awake and/or frustrated about not being asleep," you also don't need to know how many minutes have passed. Your sleep log only requires an estimate, not a precise count of how long you were awake during the night. Therefore, knowing the time does not help you in any way whatsoever. Checking the clock, on the other hand, is actively unhelpful. A classic experiment by Nicole Tang and colleagues found that, when people with insomnia were instructed to monitor a clock, they not only took longer to fall asleep but also overestimated how long they were awake, compared to those who were instructed to monitor a non-clock display.* This is not surprising! Watching the minutes slip by makes you anxious and frustrated, warping your sense of time and exacerbating your hyperarousal. Some patients have asked, "What if I still keep my alarm clock in the room and just try not to look at it?" Another study has shown that, on an involuntary level, people with insomnia have attention bias to clocks—this means they have a harder time tearing their attention away from those middle-of-the-night time displays than the average person, as if those glaring numbers are yelling at them to get their attention.† Don't keep feeding in to this! Just put the clock or phone across the room and cover it up with a T-shirt so it doesn't even tempt you to look at it.

---

* Nicole KY Tang, D. Anne Schmidt, and Allison G. Harvey, "Sleeping with the Enemy: Clock Monitoring in the Maintenance of Insomnia," *Journal of Behavior Therapy and Experimental Psychiatry* 38, no. 1 (2007): 40–55.

† H. Woods, L. M. Marchetti, S. M. Biello, and C. A. Espie, "The Clock as a Focus of Selective Attention in Those with Primary Insomnia: An Experimental Study Using a Modified Posner Paradigm," *Behaviour Research and Therapy* 47, no. 3 (2009): 231–36. https://doi.org/10.1016/J.BRAT.2008.12.009.

What to Do This Upcoming Week

First, let's briefly review your chapter 8 work on examining your unhelpful thoughts about insomnia. How has that been going? Is it easy to identify your automatic thoughts about sleep? Are they helpful thoughts? Do the pocket Socrates questions help you examine the unhelpful thoughts so you can arrive at a more accurate and fair perspective? If all of this felt too difficult, one of these things might be happening:

Your Mind Is Stuck on a Thought That Is Just *True*

A lot of your unhelpful thoughts may very well be true, or have an element of truth in them. For example, perhaps it feels frustratingly true that you *will* be tired tomorrow, because you're always tired. Fair enough! You don't need to convince yourself that you won't be tired. But the goal here isn't to magically turn a negative thought into a positive one. That's called bullshitting. Instead, we're here to stop the spiral of an unhelpful thought making you feel even worse. Ask yourself, "What if this thought is going to be true and I will be tired tomorrow? What bad consequences will come of it? How likely is the worst-case scenario? Can I cope with it?" When we respond to a vague sense of doom with concrete answers, it usually feels less bad, and we usually have a better grasp of the full truth.

You Have Trouble Coming Up with More Optimistic Thoughts

Again, we don't have to put on rose-colored glasses when approaching sleep-related thoughts. It's okay if you're not a naturally optimistic thinker. We're just trying to look at the whole picture and be fairer in our statement. Sometimes this means completing the sentence with "and . . ." For example, instead of, "I've wasted so many hours because of insomnia over the years," we can complete the sentence and say, "I've wasted so many hours because of insomnia over the years, *and* I look forward to wasting fewer from now on as my relationship with sleep continues to improve."

This Exercise Is Just Making You Struggle More with Sleep-Related Thoughts

Yup. This sometimes happens. At times, I find myself digging deeper into a debate with myself about some irksome thought, and I end up spending even more time with it. This approach of examining your thoughts is meant to offer an easy, painless path to *less* angst. If it's just making you more confused or frustrated . . . let's just drop it. Don't worry that this approach didn't work well for you. Instead, switch gears to the current chapter's "stop the struggle" approach.

Transitioning Out of the Big Reset

By now, the Big Reset should have done its job in resetting your sleep physiology. By increasing your sleep drive and decreasing all sorts of arousal, you should be seeing from your sleep logs that you're taking less time to fall asleep or fall back to sleep, on average, and having less frequent bouts of long wakefulness during the night. Your sleep efficiency should be above 85 percent on most nights, and in the 85 percent to 95 percent range on average. It's possible that these numbers haven't changed much for a few weeks, either because your numbers were already decent to begin with or because some other perpetuating factors for chronic insomnia are at work. Either way, now it's time to transition out of boot camp mindset and into sustainable mindset. This means loosening up "rules," trusting your body's signals, and letting go of rigid routines. In practice, this means:

- As long as you still keep your rise time fairly consistent (within approximately one hour), you can go to bed when you feel sleepy, instead of waiting until a planned bedtime. You'll find that this naturally falls at around the same time on most evenings.

- You can linger in bed a little in the mornings if you enjoy this. Feel free to allow yourself a snooze or a leisurely lying-in. Still get out of bed within half an hour of waking and get a dose of sunlight as soon as you can.

- You can take a regular nap if desired. I'd recommend keeping it short (set a timer for about thirty minutes, no more than an hour), and keeping it at around the same time each day, early in the afternoon so it doesn't borrow too much sleep drive from bedtime.

- You can forget to do the sleep log and shrug about it, unless doing it is helpful or enjoyable.

As you can see, this week is all about going with the flow. However, there are some healthy guardrails that I strongly encourage you to keep:

- **Continue with your light + movement routine**. Hopefully, this feels good and becomes its own reward. If not, review chapter 6 and make sure you're capturing the spirit of having fun with it.

- **Prioritize daytime rest.** Friendly reminder: Rest is not the same thing as sleep. In fact, rest often involves getting up and doing something. Deliberately plan times to engage in pleasure, daydreaming, walking, and other nonproductive activities that nourish your body and soul.

- **Practice acceptance and mindfulness.** Using the approaches outlined in this chapter, stop struggling with sleep. I especially recommend practicing the "get out of your head and into your body" exercises daily. They only take a few minutes!

BOTTOM LINE

Sleep effort is a big perpetuator of chronic insomnia. Working really hard to fall asleep or become a better sleeper often backfires by increasing hyperarousal. Instead of working harder, letting go of the struggle might just be a game changer. Stop flailing in quicksand and do these things instead:

1. **Accept reality.** Notice all the ways your mind is trying to deny or change reality. Sometimes this is disguised as overanalyzing. Take a breath. Now, say out loud what the reality is.

2. **Ask: What would a good sleeper do?** Using an effortlessly good sleeper that you know as a role model, ask what they would do in this situation and act accordingly. Send the signal to your body that insomnia isn't an ever-present threat, so it feels safe to relax.

3. **Get out of your head and into your body.** Using the mini mindfulness practices in this chapter (the 5–4–3–2–1, the mindful breath, and the body scan), practice getting grounded in reality in a nonjudgmental way. This is your most powerful tool for stopping the struggle.

4. **Stop checking the clock at night.** There is no universe in which this is helpful, so just save yourself the angst and cover up the clock with a T-shirt and put the phone across the room.

Trusting Sleep

How to Get Off Sleep Medications

A good relationship is built on trust. If you've struggled with insomnia for a while, it might be hard to trust your sleep to be there for you or to take care of you. In fact, many of my patients say that they feel like sleep has betrayed them. But you've been working on rebuilding a good relationship with sleep: using the Big Reset to make a clean slate, shifting your thinking about sleep to be fairer, and learning to let go of unhelpful sleep effort. Now may be the time to consider if you're ready for a trust fall: sleeping without medications.

Don't worry. I'm not here to call sleep medications the devil or to push you to get off them. For many people, there are very good reasons why medication is the best option. But I know from years of working with insomnia patients that, chances are, you've already been impatient to get off your sleeping pills (or your doctor has been impatient for you to do so). In this chapter, we will take a no-pressure walk through some common questions people have about insomnia medications and whether or how to get off them, to help you consider whether you're ready for the next step in your relationship with sleep.

People tend to have three big questions when it comes to sleep medications:

1. What are sleep medications, and do they work?
2. Should I start or keep taking sleep medications?
3. How do I get off them?

I'll answer all three questions in this chapter, plus another question that people don't ask, but should:

4. What is the psychology of taking sleep medications, and why is understanding this crucial for my relationship with sleep?

What Are Sleep Medications, and Do They Work?

Let's start with a brief overview of sleep medications that people take for insomnia. Please do not use this as a comprehensive guide to which medications you personally should or shouldn't take, which is a decision you should only make with your doctor and healthcare providers.* Generally, there are three categories of substances people use to try to improve insomnia:

1. FDA-approved medications that are specifically indicated for insomnia treatment
2. FDA-approved medications that are used "off-label" for insomnia treatment
3. Over-the-counter sleep aids (e.g., vitamins, supplements, herbs) that are marketed as insomnia treatments

---

* This disclaimer is especially important to heed because my expertise and credentials do *not* include medication prescribing. I have a PhD in clinical psychology, and I specialize in *behavioral* sleep medicine. Again, please talk to your doctor about medications.

In my mind, there's an unofficial fourth category: alcohol, recreational drugs, and black-market prescription medications. People use them to self-medicate, which no healthcare provider would condone as an insomnia treatment. We'll cover them in detail in chapter 11. Here, we'll focus on the first three categories.

FDA-Approved Drugs for Insomnia

These include,* in alphabetical order:

- Doxepin
- Eszopiclone
- Ramelteon
- Suvorexant
- Temazepam
- Triazolam
- Zaleplon
- Zolpidem

This list represents a remarkably diverse group of chemicals. Some are benzodiazepines (e.g., temazepam), a group of drugs that work by amplifying your brain's GABA (gamma-aminobutyric acid) system—a system that generally inhibits other brain activity. Some are marketed as "nonbenzodiazepines" (e.g., zolpidem), because benzodiazepines have a bad reputation for potential cognitive impairment side effects, as well as having potential for dependence or abuse, and serious withdrawal symptoms if not tapered very carefully. These "nonbenzos" technically have a different chemical structure, but they actually act in the same

---

* There are more, but I'm only including the ones that were discussed in the most recent American Academy of Sleep Medicine Clinical Practice Guidelines, because they generally have the most research backing.

way as benzodiazepines in the brain, and have similar side effect profiles.* Some are orexin antagonists (e.g., suvorexant), which means they
inhibit the wake-promoting orexin system in the brain. Interestingly,
people who have narcolepsy, a debilitating disorder where they become
irresistibly sleepy during the day and can have sleep attacks, don't have
enough orexin action in the brain. Some are antidepressants (e.g., doxepin) that happen to have an antihistamine effect at a low dosage, which
also blocks wake-promoting systems. And some are melatonin receptor
agonists (e.g., ramelteon), which enhance the action of the melatonin
system, whose job is to tell the rest of the brain and body when it is
nighttime.

These medications are all FDA-approved for insomnia treatment
because they've been shown to reduce the amount of time users take
to fall asleep and/or stay awake during the night and to improve general satisfaction with sleep, compared to placebo. However, the average amount of improvement is often underwhelming. For example,
zolpidem (a.k.a. Ambien) is the most commonly prescribed insomnia
medication, and its average effect on sleep latency is to reduce it by five
to twelve minutes, and the total increase in sleep duration throughout
the night is less than thirty minutes.† These numbers refer to actual
amounts of sleep change observed in the clinical trials, as measured by
polysomnography (i.e., overnight sleep study). If you feel like your Ambien increases your sleep by a lot more than a few minutes, that may be
true, or it may be due to this medication's known retrograde amnesic

* Jennifer Glass, Krista L. Lanctôt, Nathan Herrmann, Beth A. Sproule, and Usoa E Busto, "Sedative Hypnotics in Older People with Insomnia: Meta-Analysis of Risks and Benefits," *BMJ: British Medical Journal*
331, no. 7526 (2005): 1169. https://doi.org/10.1136/BMJ.38623.768588.47.

† Michael J. Sateia, Daniel J. Buysse, Andrew D. Krystal, David N. Neubauer, and Jonathan L. Heald, "Clinical Practice Guideline for the Pharmacologic Treatment of Chronic Insomnia in Adults: An American
Academy of Sleep Medicine Clinical Practice Guideline," *Journal of Clinical Sleep Medicine* 13, no. 2 (2017):
307. https://doi.org/10.5664/JCSM.6470.

effects. In other words, when you take Ambien, you may not remember being awake during the night as much as you do without the drug.

Fortunately, most of these FDA-approved insomnia medications have mild side effects and little potential harm for most people. The general expert consensus is that their benefits outweigh the risks. But one thing that surprised me when researching this category of insomnia medications is that even though AASM recommends them for treating insomnia, *none* of them received more than a "Weak" recommendation. This means that experts, upon reviewing all available data, felt there was a "lower degree of certainty in the outcome and appropriateness . . . [based on] the strength of evidence in published data." This is in contrast to a hypothetical "Strong" recommendation, which "clinicians should, under most circumstances, follow." For context, cognitive behavioral therapy for insomnia (CBT-I), which is the core approach included in the Hello Sleep program, received a "Strong" recommendation from both AASM* and the American College of Physicians.†

Why did your healthcare provider prescribe you one of these medications instead of CBT-I? It's not their fault. My colleagues in primary care, psychiatry, and neurology are the ones seeing the vast majority of patients with insomnia, and they often lament that there simply aren't any behavioral sleep medicine providers to refer their patients to. Or if their hospital system has that highly coveted CBT-I practitioner, their waiting list is months long. The fact is that there is a tremendous shortage of behavioral sleep medicine specialists, with only a couple of hundred in the *world*, mostly concentrated in the United States, and not even in every

* Jack D. Edinger, J. Todd Arnedt, Suzanne M. Bertisch, Colleen E. Carney, John J. Harrington, Kenneth L. Lichstein, Michael J. Sateia, et al., "Behavioral and Psychological Treatments for Chronic Insomnia Disorder in Adults: An American Academy of Sleep Medicine Clinical Practice Guideline." *Journal of Clinical Sleep Medicine* 17, no. 2 (2021): 255–62. https://doi.org/10.5664/jcsm.8986.

† Amir Qaseem, Devan Kansagara, Mary Ann Forciea, Molly Cooke, and Thomas D. Denberg, "Management of Chronic Insomnia Disorder in Adults: A Clinical Practice Guideline from the American College of Physicians," *Annals of Internal Medicine* 165, no. 2 (2016): 125. https://doi.org/10.7326/M15-2175.

state. Many more healthcare providers are being trained in CBT-I, but there are still not enough to go around.

Doctors and other prescribers also feel a lot of pressure to relieve their patients' insomnia symptoms quickly, because these patients are often very distressed (understandably!) about not sleeping well, sometimes even arriving at the emergency department with urgent need. When the overall healthcare system is not designed to emphasize behavioral health or preventive care, and doctors aren't able to spend more than a few minutes with their patients, the only viable option, often, is to prescribe medication. Many of my medical colleagues are reluctant to prescribe insomnia drugs long term, but between the physiological and psychological dependence that often develop once a patient starts, it never quite feels like the right time to stop. For some, the catalyst for finally trying to get off sleep aids comes when the patient turns sixty-five, and the doctor is no longer willing to keep prescribing medications that increase their risk for memory impairment, falls, and car accidents.*

SAFETY WARNING: DON'T EVER STOP TAKING BENZODIAZEPINES COLD TURKEY

All medication changes should be approved by your prescribing doctor first, but it's especially important that you never abruptly stop taking or reduce the dosage of benzodiazepines. These include: alprazolam (Xanax), diazepam (Valium), lorazepam (Ativan), clonazepam (Klonopin), and others (please double-check if your sleep medication is a benzodiazepine). Withdrawal symptoms from these medications can be deadly if they're not tapered very gradually and with close monitoring from your

---

* Glenna Brewster, Barbara Riegel, and Philip R Gehrman, "Insomnia in the Older Adult," *Sleep Medicine Clinics* 13, no. 1 (2018): 13. https://doi.org/10.1016/J.JSMC.2017.09.002.

doctor. It's sometimes difficult to gauge how "gradual" is a slow enough pace with these medications, so do NOT use the example taper schedules later in this chapter as a prescription for how to taper from your benzodiazepine.

FDA-Approved Off-Label Insomnia Drugs

These include:*

- Clonazepam
- Gabapentin
- Hydroxyzine
- Olanzapine
- Quetiapine
- Tiagabine
- Trazodone

This is an interesting category because, in a way, anything that has a sedating effect could be used off-label, which means the drug is not designed to treat insomnia, but it's prescribed for this purpose anyway. From my discussions with medical colleagues, it seems that this happens mostly because doctors are reluctant to prescribe on-label medications that have risky side effect profiles (e.g., benzodiazepines), or because their patient has already tried multiple "on-label" medications for insomnia that did not help, so now they have to get more creative. Perhaps that's why almost half the time when someone receives a prescription for insomnia, it's for an off-label drug.[†]

---

* For this list, I'm including ones that are reviewed in the latest AASM Clinical Practice Guidelines, plus a few more that I commonly see in the clinic.

† L. Leanne Lai, Mooi Heong Tan, and Yen Chi Lai, "Prevalence and Factors Associated with Off-Label

Here, again, we have a diverse group of drugs that range from anti-depressants (e.g., trazodone), to antipsychotics (e.g., quetiapine), to anti-convulsants (e.g., gabapentin). The AASM does not recommend *any* of the drugs listed above for treating insomnia, because there is either not enough evidence supporting their efficacy or that the evidence shows the harms outweigh the benefits, which might surprise you if you are among the 1 percent of the total adult population who take trazodone for insomnia.* But to be fair to your prescribing healthcare provider, they do this because trazodone often stands out as one of the least risky drugs they can give you for insomnia, especially if you're nearing retirement age or older. By the way, 1 percent may not seem like a high percentage at first glance, but consider that it represents millions of people taking a medication that is not meant to treat insomnia and not recommended for use in insomnia.

Another reason for prescribing an off-label drug for insomnia is if it better fits the patient's overall needs. If you have depression *and* insomnia, for example, your psychiatrist might prescribe a sedating antidepressant to address two birds with one stone. Please don't think that your doctor *shouldn't* be prescribing you off-label drugs, since there are many factors to consider.

Over-the-Counter Sleep Aids

These include:

- Acetaminophen
- Diphenhydramine

Antidepressant Prescriptions for Insomnia," *Drug, Healthcare and Patient Safety* 3, no. 1 (2011): 27. https://doi.org/10.2147/DHPS.S21079.

* Suzanne M. Bertisch, Shoshana J. Herzig, John W. Winkelman, and Catherine Buettner, "National Use of Prescription Medications for Insomnia: NHANES 1999–2010," *Sleep* 37, no. 2 (2014): 343–49. https://doi.org/10.5665/SLEEP.3410.

- Doxylamine
- Melatonin
- L-tryptophan
- Valerian
- Other supplements and herbs

Products in this category of sleep aids often have catchy names like Tylenol PM or ZzzQuil. Some patients feel less worried about taking them compared to prescription insomnia medications specifically because they're over-the-counter. In turn, they are also less likely to read dosage and warning labels, follow instructions, and discuss their use of these sleep aids with their healthcare providers.* This worries me because these medications are also not meant to be taken long term, or sometimes even short term if the insomnia has no clear cause. If you read the Tylenol PM label, for example, you'll see that it's meant for "occasional insomnia associated with minor aches and pains . . . not for use in treating sleeplessness without pain, or sleep problems that occur often." There are also risks for liver damage with long-term use, especially if combined with alcohol.

AASM's Clinical Practice Guidelines did not specifically mention acetaminophen medications like Tylenol PM, but they covered a few other popular over-the-counter sleep aids, including diphenhydramine, L-tryptophan, Valerian, and melatonin. None were recommended for treating insomnia.

The most popular of these nonrecommended sleep aids is melatonin, worth mentioning in detail because it represents a wildly successful marketing story for drug makers who increased its sales by more than 500

---

* Olufunmilola Abraham, Loren J. Schleiden, Amanda L. Brothers, and Steven M. Albert, "Managing Sleep Problems Using Non-Prescription Medications and the Role of Community Pharmacists: Older Adults' Perspectives," *International Journal of Pharmacy Practice* 25, no. 6 (2017): 438–46. https://doi.org /10.1111/IJPP.12334.

Table 1. List of Medications Used to Aid Sleep

MEDICATION	FDA-APPROVED SPECIFICALLY FOR INSOMNIA?	RECOMMENDED BY THE AASM TO TREAT INSOMNIA?*
BENZODIAZEPINE HYPNOTICS		
Estazolam	Yes	No Stance
Flurazepam	Yes	No Stance
Quazepam	Yes	No Stance
Temazepam	Yes	Yes
Triazolam	Yes	Yes
NONBENZODIAZEPINE HYPNOTICS		
Eszopiclone	Yes	Yes
Zaleplon	Yes	Yes
Zolpidem	Yes	Yes
BARBITURATES		
Butabarbital	Yes	No Stance
Secobarbital	Yes	No Stance
ANTIDEPRESSANTS		
Doxepin	Yes	Yes
Trazodone	No	No
OREXIN RECEPTOR ANTAGONISTS		
Suvorexant	Yes	Yes
Lemborexant	Yes	No Stance
MELATONIN RECEPTOR AGONISTS		
Ramelteon	Yes	Yes
Tasimelteon	No	No Stance
ANTIPSYCHOTICS		
Quetiapine	No	No Stance
Olanzapine	No	No Stance

ANTICONVULSANTS		
Clonazepam	No	No Stance
Gabapentin	No	No Stance
Tiagabine	No	No
ANTIHISTAMINES		
Hydroxyzine	No	No Stance
OVER-THE-COUNTER SLEEP AIDS		
Acetaminophen	No	No Stance
Diphenhydramine	Yes	No
Doxylamine	Yes	No Stance
Melatonin	No	No
L-tryptophan	No	No
Valerian	No	No
Other supplements and herbs	No	No Stance

*Based on the most recent Clinical Practice Guidelines published by the American Academy of Sleep Medicine (AASM). Yes = AASM recommends this medication for treatment of insomnia. No = AASM recommends against using this medication for treatment of insomnia. No Stance = this medication was not mentioned in the Clinical Practice Guidelines.

percent from 2003 to 2014, despite being prescription-only in the European Union and several other countries.* In the United States, where one can easily purchase it without a prescription, it's concerning how little it is regulated. For example, it's been found that the amount of melatonin contained in the pills ranged up to five times the amount declared on the label, and 26 percent of the products also contained serotonin when they're not

---

* Madeleine M. Grigg-Damberger, and Dessislava Ianakieva, "Poor Quality Control of Over-the-Counter Melatonin: What They Say Is Often Not What You Get," *Journal of Clinical Sleep Medicine* 13, no. 2 (2017): 163. https://doi.org/10.5664/JCSM.6434.

supposed to.* Most clinical trials of melatonin used dosages of two milli-grams (mg) or less, so when you're taking an over-the-counter melatonin product labeled "5 mg," you're possibly taking a pill that's many times more potent than what has been studied and deemed safe.

An even bigger issue is that many patients, through no fault of their own, misunderstand what melatonin actually does. The over-the-counter product is advertised as a sleep aid, and people expect it to have a sedating effect, but melatonin is not a sedative. It's actually a hormone, naturally produced in our brains as part of the circadian system, fluc-tuating over the twenty-four-hour day-night cycle in a natural rhythm (and also in response to how much light there is in the environment), helping our bodies to tell when it's time to sleep versus wake. This is why sleep specialists suggest that their patients use melatonin (at very low doses) four to six hours before bedtime because it helps people with delayed sleep phase disorder (i.e., severe night owls) simulate an earlier evening, so they can sleep *and wake* earlier. However, timing is import-ant when taking melatonin, because taking it in the wrong part of your twenty-four-hour cycle could shift your sleep timing *later.* In any case, it's meant to change the *timing* of your sleep, not to help you sleep lon-ger or fall asleep faster.† This means that taking melatonin at bedtime may be completely useless if your body has already been ramping up melatonin levels for several hours, or in some cases, might even backfire by making you fall asleep later or wake up earlier. That being said, it has very little potential for physiological dependency or adverse effects,

---

* Lauren A. E. Erland, and Praveen K. Saxena, "Melatonin Natural Health Products and Supplements: Presence of Serotonin and Significant Variability of Melatonin Content," *Journal of Clinical Sleep Medicine : JCSM : Official Publication of the American Academy of Sleep Medicine* 13, no. 2 (2017): 275. https://doi.org /10.5664/JCSM.6462.

† Melatonin is also used to treat other circadian rhythm sleep-wake disorders (see chapter 16) and other sleep problems like REM sleep behavior disorder.

so there's little reason to be worried about safety if you've already been taking melatonin.

Please remember that there are many, many factors to consider in whether, how, and when you take any medication. What I told you above about melatonin does not necessarily mean that it's bad and that nobody should take it. For example, pediatric experts support using it for children with autism spectrum disorders because it promotes better sleep and daytime functioning for this group.* Adults with hypertension who are treated with beta-blockers can experience decreased melatonin (and resulting insomnia) as a side effect, and for them, taking melatonin does appear to significantly improve sleep.† All of this is to say that I highly recommend consulting with your doctor about over-the-counter sleep aids even though you technically don't need their approval to buy them.

And just a last word on over-the-counter sleep aids, because I know there will be readers eagerly wondering, "What about St. John's Wort? Or kava kava?" There is simply not enough evidence to support the use of these herbs and supplements for insomnia. It's possible that one of them is a miracle cure and scientists have simply neglected to research it, but this is highly unlikely for two reasons:

1. Pharmaceutical companies are leaving no stones unturned when it comes to sleep aids. Consider how much money they stand to make if they can demonstrate that a "natural" remedy truly works for insomnia, or patent a chemical that mimics it!

---

* Carmen M. Schroder, Tobias Banaschewski, Joaquin Fuentes, Catherine Mary Hill, Allan Hvolby, Maj-Britt Posserud, and Oliviero Bruni, "Pediatric Prolonged-Release Melatonin for Insomnia in Children and Adolescents with Autism Spectrum Disorders," *Expert Opinion on Pharmacotherapy* 22, no. 18 (2021): 2445–2454.

† Frank A. J. L. Scheer, Christopher J. Morris, Joanna I. Garcia, Carolina Smales, Erin E. Kelly, Jenny Marks, Atul Malhotra, and Steven A. Shea, "Repeated Melatonin Supplementation Improves Sleep in Hypertensive Patients Treated with Beta-Blockers: A Randomized Controlled Trial," *Sleep* 35, no. 10 (2012): 1395–1402. https://doi.org/10.5665/SLEEP.2122.

If this miracle herb existed, you would certainly have tried it before buying this book.

2. We already know that chronic insomnia is driven by the way we act and think about sleep, which is why behavioral treatments work. No herb, or any medication, could plausibly take away conditioned arousal or give you sleep drive.

Should I Start or Keep Taking Insomnia Drugs?

Despite the less-than-promising evidence I've shown you above about insomnia drugs' efficacy, I'm not here to tell you that they are the devil. In fact, there are ever safer and potentially more efficacious insomnia drugs being developed, and there are people for whom one of these medications is the best option. Even if behavioral treatment were available to every single person with insomnia, there are certainly still some people who will respond better to a medication, and there is nothing wrong with that. But in my clinical experience, most people would prefer to not take sleep medication long term if possible, or their healthcare provider is increasingly reluctant to write a prescription for one as they get into retirement age.

If this is the case for you, I very much understand your dilemma—it probably doesn't feel like you have a real choice about whether to keep taking your insomnia medication, since the options seem to include only those that are bad and worse. Patients often tell me, in a resigned voice, that they'll just have to risk having memory impairment later in life, or that they just have to keep putting up with feeling hungover in the mornings. Sometimes they realize that a big part of why they feel tired during the day is not because they didn't sleep enough, but rather because their sleep medication has not yet fully left their system. Sometimes, they have tried unsuccessfully to quit sleep medications, but then turned back to them after a few sleepless nights "scared them straight."

I'm here to reassure you that, even if it doesn't feel like it right now, you hold the power to decide whether you'd like to take sleep medications or not. But don't go it alone. I strongly caution you not to make any changes to your medication, whether that's changing the dose, frequency, or timing, without your prescriber's approval. For example, it's possible that what you're being prescribed for insomnia is also serving double-duty to treat something else, such as depression, anxiety, or chronic pain. In this case, the best treatment plan overall may be to stay on this medication, or perhaps to switch to a similar but nonsedating medication, or adjust the dosage or timing . . . all with consultation with your prescriber.

What Is the Psychology Behind Taking Sleep Medications?

Whatever decision you and your doctor make together, it's helpful to be aware of the way you currently think and feel about sleep medications. This is what I mean: sleep medications aren't taken (or avoided) in a totally rational vacuum. Whether it's over-the-counter herbs or benzodiazepines or antipsychotics, and whether you're contemplating starting something or have already been taking it for twenty years, I bet the decision is not as simple as the way you think about your daily allergy medication or your once-in-a-while antibiotics.

In fact, the act of taking sleep medications is psychological. I don't mean that it's a placebo effect (although a lot of it is*), but the way we think and act around them plays a big role in our relationship with sleep. For example, if you've ever experienced any of the following, there are strong psychological forces at work in your relationship with sleep and sleep medications:

---

* W. Vaughn McCall, Ralph D'Agostino, and Aaron Dunn, "A Meta-Analysis of Sleep Changes Associated with Placebo in Hypnotic Clinical Trials," *Sleep Medicine* 4, no. 1 (2003): 57–62. https://doi.org/10.1016/S1389-9457(02)00242-3.

- You've debated at bedtime, or in the middle of the night, whether you should just say "screw it" and take that pill, but you felt guilty because you want to take it only if absolutely necessary.
- You've agonized, maybe for months, about whether getting some consistent sleep with your pill is worth the scary cognitive impairment risks that have been associated with it.
- You split your sleep pill in half (or, in the case of one patient I saw, into precise one-eighths).
- You've tried more than one brand of melatonin, just in case it makes a difference.
- You've been disappointed by valerian root, magnesium, and various supplements, but maybe you just haven't found quite the right combination yet, so you keep looking for the "right" cocktail.
- You've tried unsuccessfully to stop taking sleep medications or supplements for sleep.
- You flipped straight to this section of the book without reading chapters 1–9 first.

All these behaviors are clues that sleep medications play an outsized role in your life (even if you're not taking any!), and that this may be *contributing to your ongoing insomnia.* How? Well, remember the concept of *sleep effort* from chapter 9? Doing the "should I, or shouldn't I" dance with your sleep medication is one of the best examples of sleep effort, because it forces you to make on-the-fly decisions leading up to bedtime (or in the middle of the night) about whether and how much to take, to try to somehow quantify the benefit versus risk of a drug that you probably resent taking, and to deal with the guilt and shame that comes with feeling dependent on something. All of this angst increases—you guessed it!—arousal, making it more difficult to sleep. In the grander scheme of things, it also gives insomnia a bigger spotlight in your life overall.

The PRN Paradox

To see a concrete example of how the psychology of sleep medications may be keeping you stuck in insomnia, let's take a look at the powerful PRN paradox.

Whatever you're taking for sleep, I'll bet that your doctor prescribed it "PRN," which stands for pro re nata, Latin for "as the need arises." This means that your sleeping pill was not meant to be taken every night, indefinitely, the way blood pressure medications are to be taken . . . at least not for more than a couple of weeks in a row. Rather, you're encouraged to take your sleeping pill only as needed and only for a short period.

This puts the burden on you to figure out what "as needed" means and how long is too long to keep taking the drug, which pours more fuel on the insomnia fire. Now, not only are you treating sleep as an upcoming battle, but you're tiptoeing around the sleeping pill itself as if it were dangerous, further raising alarms and jacking up arousal.

Put another way: Let's say your friend invites you to a party. She tells you that it's just a casual, low-key get-together at her sister's place and should be a relaxed affair. But you see that she's agonizing over what she should wear, meticulously arranging fancy appetizers to bring, studying blueprints of her sister's house, and packing brass knuckles in her purse while nervously muttering, "Just in case." How would this make you feel? Confused, perhaps. Nervous, certainly. Are you going to happy hour or joining bizarro fight club?

This is what's happening to your brain when you overthink your sleep medications. You're trying to convince your mind and body to chill out about sleep, but all the mental gymnastics about whether and when and how often and what dosage of your Ambien to take is giving all your systems the opposite of relaxing signals. With all this preparation and strategizing, you're clearly preparing for D-Day. Even if you don't agonize over sleep medications in such a dramatic way, having a low-simmering, chronic indecision about sleep medications can similarly strain your relationship with sleep.

You may be thinking, "Well, that's why I want to take sleep medication as little as possible. I don't want to become dependent on it. In fact, I only take my Lunesta when I *really* need it, and even then, I try to only take half a pill."

But what does "really need it" mean? When you've been awake for one hour? Two hours? When you haven't slept well for three nights in a row? Or four nights? Or four nights this week, not necessarily in a row? What if you already took a full pill last night? Half pill? What if you already took Benadryl earlier? If you're trying really hard to cut down on your sleep meds but find yourself bargaining or unwilling to totally let go . . . I'm sorry, but you're *already* psychologically dependent.

In other words, trying to minimize your dependence on sleep medications by using it "as needed" often backfires. It makes sleep into a math problem, sinking you deeper into chronic insomnia. And, ironically, this makes it harder to get off sleep medications.

Pills Get False Credit

Another powerful psychological force is misattribution, which means assigning blame and credit to the wrong things, such as thanking your lucky hat for your team's Super Bowl win. If you've ever tried to stop taking your sleep medications, or have tried intermittent dosing (a.k.a. only taking it after having had X number of bad nights in a row), you may have already experienced misattribution.

It may have gone something like this: You read an article about how Ambien can increase risk for cognitive problems, so you resolve to get off it. You're feeling anxious because you've been taking it for a long time, and you're not at all confident that you can sleep well without it.

(Not to mention you're also wondering if you've doomed yourself to dementia.)

Just as you predicted, you go three nights with hardly any sleep, and you're feeling as bad as you've ever felt. On the fourth night you think to yourself, "Well, not sleeping will give me dementia too. Screw it." After taking your Ambien that night, you sleep like a log for nine hours straight. You resign yourself to the lesser of two evils because now you have proof that you can't sleep without Ambien.

This chain of events and thinking is *so* understandable. In any situation other than insomnia, I would have done the same. But it doesn't have to go like this. Let's break it down:

- Coming off sleep medications cold turkey, especially prescription-only ones like Ambien, will certainly lead to a temporary increase in insomnia. This is called "rebound insomnia," which is a common withdrawal symptom. Your body is reacting to the sudden absence of a chemical it has come to expect.
- After this happens for a few days, you may become legitimately sleep-deprived, just as you would be if you pulled three all-nighters in a row to study for an exam. What happens when we stay up for a very long time, and sleep very little? Our sleep drive accumulates until our piggy bank is overflowing. On the fourth night, all this sleep drive finally overwhelms our body's withdrawal reaction, and we get to sleep heavily.
- BUT, from your perspective, it's not your sleep drive that's finally putting you to sleep. It's that "screw it" pill you finally caved in and took on the fourth night. Hence, misattribution. You've given credit to the medication for making you sleep when it was really your own sleep drive's work.
- Not only have you given credit to the wrong source, but you've also given yourself "proof" that you cannot sleep without the

medication. But that's not true! I could create rebound insomnia in even a lifelong good sleeper by giving them Ambien for a couple of weeks and then suddenly taking it away. The temporary rebound insomnia is a physiological reaction that goes away with time.

How to Come Off Sleep Medications

The good news is if you want to come off sleep medications, the process is actually pretty straightforward. In fact, it might be one of the easier things in this book to do.

I remember one motivated patient named Paul who called me on January 2, 2019. He said that his number one goal for the year was to come off his cocktail of sleep aids, including a half-dozen over-the-counter supplements and one Ambien prescription. He said he had tried to quit multiple times before without success, but this time he meant to make it stick, so he'd set aside $10,000 toward this goal. He asked if I thought his timeline and budget were reasonable. Three months and a couple of hundred dollars in copays later, he was medication-free (and planning a $9,800 vacation to Europe).

Just because you've tried to come off sleep medications before without success doesn't mean you can't do it now. You just need some science-based guidance and realistic reassurance. The most effective and sustainable method for getting off insomnia medications is based on three principles:

1. **Take decision-making out of the equation:** We're going to stop with the bargaining and agonizing and guilting. Instead, we're going to make your medication-taking behavior so automated and banal that you're going to almost forget that it's

a *thing*. In fact, the way Paul and many of my other patients ended up taking the final step to zero sleep medications is that they simply forgot to take them for a few nights in a row and never looked back.

2. **Do it after completing the Hello Sleep program (or an equivalent evidence-based insomnia program):** You're much likelier to succeed if you have the foundational skills and knowledge from cognitive behavioral therapy for insomnia (CBT-I) and other components of the Hello Sleep program. Having a solid relationship with sleep first, or at least being on the trajectory to having one, is like fixing your car before you start a long road trip—it will make the journey smoother and more likely to go as planned. While you're still working through Hello Sleep, you should continue taking your sleep medications on a consistent schedule (ideally, same dosage and timing every night, or at some other predictable interval).

3. **Taper off gradually:** Stopping sleep medications cold turkey is usually ineffective because rebound insomnia is so miserable. The experience of caving in after a few nights may even reinforce the idea that you can't sleep without the drug. That's why some people end up even more addicted to their sleep medication after a cold-turkey quit attempt than they were before. Also, quitting some medications cold turkey has dangerous side effects, so it's never advisable to do so without consulting your doctor.

The exact medication taper schedule is different for each person, depending on which medications they're taking, but they should follow the three principles above. For example, benzodiazepines are usually tapered much more slowly than other insomnia medications, because the withdrawal symptoms can be dangerous and debilitating.* Next, we'll walk through a couple of sample step-by-step taper schedules. Before you read further, let me emphasize, again, that you should not make any changes to your medication-taking behaviors without consulting with your prescribing provider first. They might, for example, switch you to an extended release version of what you're currently taking before tapering you off, or they may want you to taper much more gradually than the sample schedules in this book. You can show your doctor these proposed schedules to see if they approve, or if they suggest modifications.

Step-by-Step Sample Taper Plans

Tapering Off a Single Sleep Medication That You Currently Take Regularly

Sondra is prescribed to take fifty milligrams of trazodone nightly. She tries to take a half pill on most nights, and doesn't take any on approximately one night per week. But sometimes she has a particularly stressful day and takes a full pill in anticipation of having more trouble than usual with falling asleep. Sometimes, she'll take another half pill when she wakes up during the night. Here's what I would recommend for Sondra: after finishing part II (The Big Reset) and part III (Going Deeper into the Relationship) of this book:

1. Establish a consistent nightly dosage that is close to what she's already doing. Do not take any more or less than this on any given night, and absolutely no extra "rescue" doses during the night.

---

* Jonathan P. Hintze, and Jack D. Edinger, "Hypnotic Discontinuation in Chronic Insomnia," *Sleep Medicine Clinics* 15, no. 2 (2020): 147–54. https://doi.org/10.1016/J.JSMC.2020.02.003.

2. Begin taking a smaller dose on predetermined nights. Gradually decrease the dose over several weeks.

Sondra's sample week-by-week plan (Version A):

- Week 1: Take 25 mg (half a pill) every night.
- Week 2: Take 12.5 mg (one-quarter of a pill) on Tuesday and Friday. Continue taking 25 mg (half a pill) on all other nights.
- Week 3: Take 12.5 mg (one-quarter of a pill) on Monday, Tuesday, Friday, and Saturday. Continue taking 25 mg on all other nights.
- Week 4: Take 12.5 mg (one-quarter of a pill) every night.
- Week 5: Take 0 mg (no pill) on Tuesday and Friday. Continue taking 12.5 mg (one-quarter of a pill) on all other nights.
- Week 6: Skip the dose on Monday, Tuesday, Friday, and Saturday. Continue taking 12.5 mg (one-quarter of a pill) on all other nights.
- Week 7: No trazodone.

Note: The specific nights of each week when Sondra was to take a smaller dose than before were all predetermined at the very beginning of the taper plan. Once she had chosen these nights for each week of the plan, they were written in stone. She had to follow the plan regardless of how she felt on any given night and regardless of any special events going on. This took all decision-making out of the six-week process.

Sondra's sample week-by-week plan (Version B):

- Week 1: Take 25 mg (half a pill) every night.
- Week 2: Take 25 mg (half a pill) every night.
- Week 3: Take 12.5 mg (one-quarter of a pill) every night.

- Week 4: Take 12.5 mg (one-quarter of a pill) every night.
- Week 5: No trazodone.

Note: This much simpler alternative for Sondra is to simply reduce her dosage by one-quarter of a pill every one to two weeks. It goes faster but is easier to remember. Whichever version takes the most guesswork out of the plan is the better one.

If Sondra were starting out with taking a full pill (50 mg) on most nights, we'd do a similar taper plan that starts, during Week 1, with her taking a full pill every night, then going down to three-quarters of a pill, then half a pill, and so forth.

Tapering Off a Single Sleep Medication That You Only Occasionally Take

As he felt his sleep improving with behavioral insomnia therapy, Suheil cut down his eszopiclone use on his own. Now he's taking one to two milligrams two to three nights per week, usually on the nights before the busiest days at work. He would like to be completely medication-free. Here's what I would recommend for Suheil:

1. Establish a consistent and predetermined medication schedule close to what he is already doing. No need to increase his pill-taking frequency to every night like Sondra since he's already taking it on fewer than half the nights.
2. Cut out one dose, on a predetermined night, per week.

A sample week-by-week plan:

- Week 1: Take 1 mg on Sunday, Monday, and Wednesday
- Week 2: Take 1 mg on Sunday, Monday, and Wednesday

- Week 3: Take 1 mg on Sunday and Wednesday
- Week 4: Take 1 mg on Sunday
- Week 5: No eszopiclone

Note: You'll notice that Week 1 and Week 2 are the same. I'm just playing it safe and slow with Suheil because he was sometimes taking one milligram and sometimes two milligrams. I would rather see him stay steady on the lower dose for a couple of weeks before rocking the boat by decreasing how often he takes it. There were times when he forgot to take his eszopiclone on a scheduled night, so in those cases we just skipped that night. Don't make up a skipped night by taking it the next day, and again, don't take any "rescue" doses in the middle of the night.

Tapering Off Multiple Sleep Aids

Paul takes ten milligrams of zolpidem on most nights. He also takes a ten-milligram melatonin gummy, over-the-counter magnesium, zinc, valerian, ashwagandha extract, and L-tryptophan. He follows a precise routine of taking these seven sleep aids nightly. He feels more confident about his sleep now after completing the first four sessions of one-on-one insomnia therapy, and would like to see how much of his "cocktail" he can cut out. Here's what I would recommend for Paul:

1. Start by cutting out the sleep aids that he is the least attached to, one at a time. Since none of the over-the-counter sleep aids he's taking are likely to make a real impact on insomnia symptoms, it doesn't matter which of them goes first.
2. When he gets down to Ambien alone, decrease the dose by five milligrams every one to two weeks.

A sample week-by-week plan:

- Week 1: Cut out L-tryptophan. Continue taking everything else.
- Week 2: Cut out valerian. Continue taking everything else.
- Week 3: Cut out zinc. Continue taking everything else.
- Week 4: Cut out ashwagandha extract. Continue taking everything else.
- Week 5: Cut out magnesium. Continue taking everything else.
- Week 6: Cut out melatonin. Continue taking 15 mg of Ambien nightly.
- Week 7: Take 10 mg Ambien on all nights.
- Week 8: Take 10 mg Ambien on all nights.
- Week 9: Take 5 mg Ambien on all nights.
- Week 10: Take 5 mg Ambien on all nights.
- Week 11: No Ambien.

Note: In reality, Paul hesitated when it came to Week 6 because he felt strongly that melatonin was helping him and was reluctant to cut it out so abruptly, so we tweaked the plan and allowed him melatonin on every other night first (while still taking the Ambien), before cutting it out completely in Week 7. He was surprised that this made no difference in his sleep, and gained more confidence in the taper plan. He ended up skipping Week 10 because he simply forgot to take his Ambien for a few nights in a row and decided to not look back.

We did make sure that at every step of tapering down Ambien, Paul felt ready to move forward, because it's better to linger at a dosage for a week or two longer than planned than to backtrack to a higher dosage. So, we took our time getting to zero Ambien.

If you are taking multiple prescription sleep medications, consult with your prescriber to decide which one to taper first. I recommend starting with the over-the-counter ones, or the medications that are less likely to cause withdrawal symptoms, and only working on tapering one at a time. Be patient. It's better to come off your sleep medications in a sustainable way than to go too quickly and lose confidence in the process.

TIPS FOR MINIMIZING REBOUND INSOMNIA

- Remember that this is a natural and temporary reaction. Help yourself increase sleep drive and decrease arousal using the approaches you're now familiar with. If needed, go all the way back to chapter 4 to re-do a Big Reset.
- If you don't need to do a full Big Reset, consider completing sleep logs to help yourself at least stay on track with a consistent wake time and avoiding spending too much time in bed.
- Redouble your favorite skills for decreasing arousal, such as keeping up with your light + movement routine, doing a daily mental litter box, and doing a body scan mindfulness exercise each evening.
- Do get out of bed if you find yourself wide awake or getting frustrated about not sleeping. Remember that sleep does not appreciate brute force.
- Remember how far you've already come! Hang in there and look forward to the type of relationship you'd like to have with your sleep in the long run.

BOTTOM LINE

- Sleep aids include a wide range of prescription and nonprescription medications. Some of them are FDA-approved for insomnia treatment, some are FDA-approved but used "off-label" for insomnia, and some are sold over-the-counter.

- The FDA-approved insomnia medications have demonstrated efficacy for improving nighttime insomnia symptoms, and experts generally agree that the risks outweigh the benefits for most patients.

- The American Academy of Sleep Medicine does not recommend off-label or over-the-counter medications for treating insomnia, either because they likely don't work or because their potential harms outweigh the benefits. However, your prescribing healthcare provider may have a specific and good reason for giving you an off-label drug for insomnia.

- Whether you start, change, or stop taking insomnia medications is a decision you should make with your doctor or healthcare providers.

- If you'd like to get off of insomnia medications, it's helpful to understand the psychology of taking them:

  » The PRN paradox: taking sleeping pills "as needed" instead of on a consistent schedule, which increases arousal and further strains your relationship with sleep.

  » Giving sleeping pills credit for helping you sleep, instead of giving credit to your own sleep drive, makes you psychologically dependent on these drugs.

- To taper off of insomnia medications, consult your prescriber and follow these principles:

  » Don't make on-the-fly decisions. Make a set-in-stone taper plan before you start and follow it to the letter, which will take decision-making angst out of the process and make you more likely to quit and stay quit.

  » Do the Hello Sleep program (or work with a behavioral sleep medicine specialist) first before starting your taper.

- Taper off gradually, instead of cold turkey. Some medications, such as those belonging to the benzodiazepine group, should be tapered very slowly to minimize potentially dangerous withdrawal effects.

11

···············

Tying Up Loose Ends

The Facts on Screens, Coffee, and Other
Sleep Hygiene Topics

A few years ago, I found myself giving opposite advice to two back-to-back insomnia patients in my Wednesday clinic at Duke. The 9:00 A.M. patient, Keisha, was a conscientious young woman who, as a former professional athlete, thrived on self-discipline. By the time she came to see me, she had cut out all caffeine and alcohol from her life, never turned on an electronic device after 9:00 P.M., and avoided exercising in the evening—all for the sake of better sleep hygiene. The 10:00 A.M. patient, Wei, was an extroverted young man who had recently ended a long-term romantic relationship and found himself "without guardrails in his routine" (his own words). He was playing video games and trading cryptocurrency late into the evening, and often going out drinking more than he intended to on weekends.

Here's what I said to Keisha: "Girl, live your life. Enjoy your coffee and alcohol and *Great British Baking Show* marathons. Depriving yourself of these little pleasures is actually exacerbating your insomnia because it's sleep effort."

Here's what I said to Wei: "Let's consider adding some guardrails back into your life. How would you feel about an evening screen curfew and some goals for reducing alcohol consumption?"

The reason I wrote off sleep hygiene with Keisha, but ultimately spent multiple sessions emphasizing it with Wei, is because substances and screens played very different roles in their relationships with sleep. For Keisha, whatever potential amount of sleep detriment she might get from a little bit of caffeine or evening light was nothing compared to the unhelpful arousal she was experiencing from her sleep effort. For Wei, although sleep drive and arousal were still the main perpetuating factors of his insomnia, his evening activities were getting in the way of fully restoring sleep health.

I tell their stories because, to be honest, I'm a little worried about putting this chapter out into the world without an opportunity to tailor the message for each reader. Later, when I describe how alcohol disrupts sleep, for example, I run the risk of giving the Keishas of the world a false impression that their sleep is so fragile that a drop of alcohol would ruin it. But I also would be remiss to not mention alcohol's effect on sleep because the Weis need to know why their sleep still doesn't feel good even though they've done great with the Big Reset. Moreover, wherever you are on the spectrum between Keisha and Wei, sleep hygiene problems are not likely the main reason for your insomnia, and I don't want you to place too much emphasis on perfecting your sleep environment or habits at the expense of doing the real work (like the Big Reset). This is why I waited until now to talk about this topic.

Here's the deal: I'll give you rigorously researched facts and my best clinical insights; you'll decide for yourself how important each of these loose-end items is for you, keeping in mind that this chapter alone will not do anything for your insomnia without the real work outlined in the previous chapters. What the tips in this chapter may do for you is to take you the rest of the way from "I'm feeling much better than before" to "I'm feeling really great." Let's start with the easy ones.

Exercising Close to Bedtime Is Perfectly fine

The advice to avoid exercising close to bedtime has been clearly debunked. Not only do we know from plenty of laboratory studies that evening exercise is not detrimental to sleep, we also know from recently published real-life data from more than 12,600 people that even moderate-to-vigorous exercise within two hours of bedtime is perfectly fine for sleep.* In fact, exercising was associated with a tiny bit more sleep and ease with falling asleep, perhaps because it is generally good for our mental and physical health, not to mention great for building up sleep drive. This is why I highly recommend that my patients exercise whenever they're able to—because between work, kids, bad weather, and lapses in motivation, it's hard enough to incorporate exercise in our lives without limiting the times of day when we're *allowed* to do it.

TV and Other Lights/Noises in the Bedroom Are Not Ideal

We know from plenty of research that reducing nighttime light and noise in hospitals improves patients' sleep.† Your home environment likely has fewer light/noise intrusions than an intensive care unit, but if

---

* Michal Kahn, Topi Korhonen, Leena Leinonen, Kaisu Martinmaki, Liisa Kuula, Anu Katriina Pesonen, and Michael Gradisar, "Is It Time We Stop Discouraging Evening Physical Activity? New Real-World Evidence From 150,000 Nights," *Frontiers in Public Health* 9 (November 2021): 1680. https://doi.org/10.3389/FPUBH.2021.772376/BIBTEX.

† Jennifer R. Dubose, and Khatereh Hadi, "Improving Inpatient Environments to Support Patient Sleep," *International Journal for Quality in Health Care* 28, no. 5 (2016): 540–53. https://doi.org/10.1093/INTQHC/MZW079.

you do have the TV on in the bedroom or a noisy household, these are relatively straightforward things to target for improving sleep. Hopefully, by now, you no longer watch TV in bed or have a TV in the bedroom at all (remember conditioned arousal?), but if watching TV at bedtime is absolutely nonnegotiable for you, I suggest these changes:

- Do most of your TV watching in another room in the evening, and try to wean off watching TV in the bedroom as much as possible.
- Set a sleep timer on your TV in the bedroom so that if you fall asleep, it will automatically turn off after a short while instead of disturbing your sleep all night.

Even without a TV in the bedroom, other sources of light (e.g., bright outdoor streetlight that shines through your window, your partner's reading lamp) may disrupt your sleep, too, by keeping you in shallower sleep and interrupting your sleep with micro wakeups.* Of course, many people can't fully control their sleeping environment, and that can be very frustrating. In those cases, I highly recommend earplugs and eye masks. These may take a little bit of getting used to, but can ultimately make a big difference. Now on to tougher topics.

Caffeine Can Be Tricky

Americans consumed almost twenty-seven million bags of coffee in the 2019–2020 fiscal year.† I don't mean the little bags you might give a co-

---

* Jounhong Ryan Cho, Eun Yeon Joo, Dae Lim Koo, and Seung Bong Hong, "Let There Be No Light: The Effect of Bedside Light on Sleep Quality and Background Electroencephalographic Rhythms," *Sleep Medicine* 14, no. 12 (2013): 1422–25. https://doi.org/10.1016/J.SLEEP.2013.09.007.

† "Coffee Consumption U.S. 2019/2020," Statista, 2021, https://www.statista.com/statistics/804271/domestic-coffee-consumption-in-the-us/.

worker for Christmas. I mean 132-pound industrial bags of coffee. I'm sure a big part of it is because we like the taste, but imagine what would happen if every Starbucks employee went on strike tomorrow. The riots will not just be about people's palates being unsatisfied. But how is this collective coffee addiction affecting us?

It is undeniable that caffeine impacts sleep. We know that, when studied systematically in the lab, **increasing doses of caffeine were increasingly bad for objectively measured sleep quantity and quality, especially if consumed close to bedtime**. The interesting thing is that if you simply ask people, they often underestimate how much caffeine affects their sleep, not noticing the more fragmented sleep, more awakenings, and decreased deep sleep.[*]

Why does caffeine affect sleep? Remember sleep drive, which we save up during the day and allows us to sleep at night? Sleep drive, on a brain chemistry level, represents the accumulation of adenosine, a by-product of energy expenditure—the more it accumulates in the brain, the more sleep drive we have. Caffeine competes with adenosine in the brain. It takes up space at the brain cell receptors where adenosine would normally dock, blocking adenosine and tricking the brain into believing that there is less of it (i.e., less sleep drive) than there is.[†] That's why, if you absolutely must stay awake after a long day, drinking coffee may help you to do so.

But caffeine is false fuel. It doesn't actually give you real energy the way nutritious food does, and it doesn't actually satisfy the need for sleep the way sleep does. That's why regularly drinking a lot of

---

[*] Ian Clark, and Hans Peter Landolt, "Coffee, Caffeine, and Sleep: A Systematic Review of Epidemiological Studies and Randomized Controlled Trials," *Sleep Medicine Reviews* 31 (February 2017): 70–78. https://doi.org/10.1016/J.SMRV.2016.01.006.

[†] Mark J. Davis, Zuowei Zhao, Howard S. Stock, Kristen A. Mehl, James Buggy, and Gregory A. Hand, "Central Nervous System Effects of Caffeine and Adenosine on Fatigue," *American Journal of Physiology-Regulatory Integrative and Comparative Physiology* 284, no. 2 (2003): 399–404. https://doi.org/10.1152/AJPREGU.00386.2002/ASSET/IMAGES/LARGE/H60231550004.JPEG.

coffee can actually make you *more* tired. It replaces the fuel that you actually need with an artificial high, forcing your body to run harder on less gas. You may also develop tolerance to caffeine over time, needing larger quantities to feel like your baseline self. And as you withdraw from caffeine in the afternoon and evening, you may experience the "crash" of fatigue even as the lingering effects of caffeine continue to block adenosine activity in the brain. Hence, the feeling of being tired but wired. And if you've been a regular coffee drinker for a while, this vicious cycle of events may seem so normal that you wouldn't even pause to consider whether caffeine is playing a role in your fatigue and insomnia.

One of the tricky things about caffeine advice is that people have a big range in their caffeine sensitivity,* so three cups of coffee per day can be totally reasonable for one person and devastating for another. How sensitive someone is depends, in part, on their genes, which dictate how we metabolize caffeine and how this affects our other chemical systems (e.g., adenosine, melatonin). It also depends on age, where middle-aged and older adults are much more sensitive than younger adults to caffeine's effects on sleep.

Of course, you're wondering, "So how much is 'too much' for *me*?" There is no consensus since there is so much variation between people. There is also wide variation in how long it takes for caffeine to leave our systems, which is why advice for how long you should abstain from caffeine before bedtime ranges anywhere from four to eleven hours.[†]

What this means for you: If you're a regular coffee drinker, and you're still feeling tired during the day even though you're sleeping

---

* Ian Clark and Hans Peter Landolt, "Coffee, Caffeine, and Sleep: A Systematic Review of Epidemiological Studies and Randomized Controlled Trials," *Sleep Medicine Reviews* 31 (February 2017): 70–78. https://doi.org/10.1016/J.SMRV.2016.01.006.

† Christopher Drake, Timothy Roehrs, John Shambroom, and Thomas Roth, "Caffeine Effects on Sleep Taken 0, 3, or 6 Hours before Going to Bed," *Journal of Clinical Sleep Medicine* 9, no. 11 (2013): 1195–1200. https://doi.org/10.5664/JCSM.3170.

better than before, try to gradually (very gradually!) reduce your caffeine intake and see what happens. Whatever amount you're consuming now, it probably doesn't hurt to eventually consume less, or to do it earlier in the day. In 2021, a study showed that quitting caffeine cold turkey for one week didn't really help poor sleepers,* but I believe this is at least partially due to reducing caffeine too suddenly. In chapter 10, we covered how to taper off of sleep medications. You can use the same principles to reduce caffeine as well.

Nicotine Is Detrimental to Sleep

People who smoke generally have a harder time with sleep and are twice as likely as nonsmokers to have significant sleep problems like insomnia and sleep apnea. In part, this is because nicotine is a stimulant, and in part because nicotine withdrawal during the night can make one wake up more often and have less REM sleep. Lung problems can also make it more difficult to breathe and sleep well at night.

I used to cofacilitate a smoking cessation group at the Veterans Administration in Boston, so I've seen firsthand the trickiness of quitting smoking when it comes to sleep. For many, they almost immediately experienced better sleep after quitting, but for others, sleep became a bigger problem (at least temporarily) when they were experiencing the withdrawal symptoms that came with it. It's already a difficult enough process, so I can understand how rocking the boat on sleep might make it even harder. If you're thinking about quitting nicotine products, I recommend working with a behavioral medicine specialist or attending a smoking cessation group. Having some social support and guidance can go a long way!

---

* Leah A. Irish, Michael P. Mead, Li Cao, Allison C. Veronda, and Ross D. Crosby, "The Effect of Caffeine Abstinence on Sleep among Habitual Caffeine Users with Poor Sleep," *Journal of Sleep Research* 30, no. 1 (2021). https://doi.org/10.1111/JSR.13048.

Alcohol, in Excess, Is Detrimental to Sleep

Even though alcohol is a sedative, it doesn't encourage good quality sleep. It might make you fall asleep faster, but as the night goes on and you experience withdrawal from alcohol, you will experience more fragmented sleep. Chronically problematic alcohol use leads to having less deep sleep and more problems with breathing during sleep.* Sadly, this also makes alcohol detox and abstinence very difficult, because many people experience significant insomnia and nightmares after quitting alcohol.†

Just as with caffeine, there is a wide range in how much alcohol affects each person. That's why there is also no universal recommendation for how much and when to drink to avoid it affecting sleep problems. There's evidence that even a small amount (one to two drinks) can somewhat affect heart rate variability during sleep,‡ but it's hard to quantify exactly how much is too much and for whom.

Here's my philosophy: If you generally have a healthy relationship with alcohol, live your life. Enjoy your wine with dinner and the occasional multi-cocktail party. Your small amount of alcohol consumption is not likely a big culprit in your sleep problems. But if you are concerned about your alcohol use or just generally want to reduce it, you can certainly use potentially better sleep as an incentive. If you currently drink alcohol specifically to help yourself fall asleep, I would

---

* Mahesh M. Thakkar, Rishi Sharma, and Pradeep Sahota, "Alcohol Disrupts Sleep Homeostasis," *Alcohol* 49, no. 4 (2015): 299–310. https://doi.org/10.1016/J.ALCOHOL.2014.07.019

† Jana Steinig, Ronja Foraita, Svenja Happe, and Martin Heinze, "Perception of Sleep and Dreams in Alcohol-Dependent Patients during Detoxication and Abstinence," *Alcohol and Alcoholism* 46, no. 2 (2011): 143–47. https://doi.org/10.1093/ALCALC/AGQ087.

‡ Julia Pietilë, Elina Helander, Ilkka Korhonen, Tero Myllymëki, Urho M. Kujala, and Harri Lindholm, "Acute Effect of Alcohol Intake on Cardiovascular Autonomic Regulation During the First Hours of Sleep in a Large Real-World Sample of Finnish Employees: Observational Study," *JMIR Mental Health* 5, no. 1 (2018). https://doi.org/10.2196/MENTAL.9519.

strongly recommend stopping this practice, because it's likely backfiring by making your sleep worse *and* increasing your angst about insomnia.

Cannabis (CBD, THC) Is Probably Not Helping Sleep

Cannabis sativa is the plant that marijuana products are made from, and it contains many chemical compounds, including cannabinoids. The most well-known cannabinoids are tetrahydrocannabinol (THC), which is the compound that gives users the desired high, and cannabidiol (CBD), which does not have psychoactive properties.[*]

Both THC and CBD interact with the brain's endocannabinoid system, which in turn has a role in the complex sleep-wake system. Based on animal studies, we know that these cannabinoids could induce sleep by increasing adenosine. However, the story may be more complicated. Cannabis consumption can indeed decrease the amount of wakefulness during the night and even increase deep sleep brain activity, but it depends on how much and what form of cannabis is used.[†] For example, higher doses of THC *increase* nighttime wakefulness and daytime sleepiness, but CBD works in the opposite direction—higher doses can increase sleep, but lower doses are associated with more insomnia. It gets more complicated: THC use can disrupt a person's circadian rhythms, which can negatively impact sleep, and withdrawal from cannabis makes sleep worse in most people.[‡] Even though people commonly believe

---

[*] National Center for Complementary and Integrative Health, "Cannabis (Marijuana) and Cannabinoids: What You Need to Know," November 2019, https://www.nccih.nih.gov/health/cannabis-marijuana-and-cannabinoids-what-you-need-to-know.

[†] Kimberly A. Babson, James Sottile, and Danielle Morabito, "Cannabis, Cannabinoids, and Sleep: A Review of the Literature," *Current Psychiatry Reports* 19, no. 4 (2017): 1–12. https://doi.org/10.1007/S11920-017-0775-9.

[‡] Karen I. Bolla, Suzanne R. Lesage, Charlene E. Gamaldo, David N. Neubauer, Nae Yuh Wang, Frank R. Funderburk, Richard P. Allen, Paula M. David, and Jean Lud Cadet, "Polysomnogram Changes in

that using cannabis helps with sleep, which it might in the very short term, long-term use is likely to backfire.* Altogether, the most recent research suggests that cannabis use, especially heavy use, is associated with poorer sleep health.†

What does this mean for you? **If you're a regular cannabis consumer (especially if THC is involved), it wouldn't hurt to reduce your intake, and you may see an improvement in sleep. But do it gradually to help minimize withdrawal symptoms. If you are not already regularly using cannabis, but are wondering whether you should start in order to help with sleep, I would recommend against it.** Not only would you be messing with a complex brain system with potentially backfiring effects for sleep, you'd also be giving yourself psychological dependence on a substance for sleep, which helps to keep insomnia going (see chapter 10).

SUMMARY ON SUBSTANCES AND SLEEP

Is consuming caffeine/nicotine/alcohol/cannabis or other recreational drugs bad for sleep?

Yes, to varying degrees. There may be specific doses of CBD or THC (both cannabinoids) that can help with sleep in the short term, but they are likely not helpful in the long term.

Marijuana Users Who Report Sleep Disturbances during Prior Abstinence," *Sleep Medicine* 11, no. 9 (2010): 882–89. https://doi.org/10.1016/J.SLEEP.2010.02.013.

* Calvin Diep, Chenchen Tian, Kathak Vachhani, Christine Won, Duminda N Wijeysundera, Hance Clarke, Mandeep Singh, and Karim S Ladha, "Recent Cannabis Use and Nightly Sleep Duration in Adults: A Population Analysis of the NHANES from 2005 to 2018," *Regional Anesthesia & Pain Medicine* 47 (December 2021): 100–104. https://doi.org/10.1136/RAPM-2021-103161.

† Kimberly A. Babson, James Sottile, and Danielle Morabito, "Cannabis, Cannabinoids, and Sleep: A Review of the Literature," *Current Psychiatry Reports* 19, no. 4 (2017): 1–12. https://doi.org/10.1007/S11920-017-0775-9.

If I do cut out all these substances, will this cure my insomnia?

No, not necessarily. Once you have addressed the core perpetuating factors of chronic insomnia (e.g., chronically low sleep drive and high arousal), reducing excessive substance use can certainly help improve sleep even more, but detoxing from all substances only is no guarantee for overcoming insomnia.

Do I need to cut out all these substances from my life to overcome insomnia?

No, not necessarily. You don't need to become a monk to overcome insomnia. For many people, it's perfectly fine for their overall sleep health to enjoy a small to moderate amount of caffeine and alcohol, for example. But remember that you may be more sensitive to caffeine than others, or it can last longer in your system, so as a habit, err on the side of consuming it less and earlier in the day. If possible, I would strongly recommend reducing or quitting nicotine.

Bed Partners (Human and Otherwise) Might Interfere with Sleep

I love to cuddle. It's one of my favorite activities. Years ago, my partner and I used to sleep with three dogs (two German Shepherds and a Lab mix) in the bed with us, and it was a very cuddly arrangement. But I was dragging myself around during the day even after nine hours of sleep, wondering what was wrong with me. Now I know better and sleep in my own room, needing significantly less sleep to feel very good during the day. Why? I believe three major things are better for my sleep now:

- Less disturbance from bed partners (human and dogs)
- Going to bed at the right time
- Better air quality

Less Disturbance from Bed Partners

You might not realize how much having another body in the bed impacts your sleep. If your partner is a healthy sleeper, you're being woken by them five and a half times per night, on average. If you have insomnia, you're waking your partner up 6.9 times per night. If your partner has obstructive sleep apnea, they're waking you up nine times *per hour*, and more if their apnea is severe. If you and your partner go to bed at the same time, you're especially likely to interrupt each other's sleep.[*] You likely don't remember most of these awakenings because they are brief, and a handful of brief awakenings are quite normal to have during a good night of sleep, but having many additional externally induced awakenings can be detrimental.

When it comes to pets, research shows that many people enjoy sharing a bed with their dog (I'm not surprised), but that even when they didn't think this disturbed their sleep, objective sleep measures found that it did. The good news is that your sleep can be better when your dog is in the room with you, but not on the bed.[†] A great compromise that my dogs and I have been happy with: we spend the night in the same room, but I sleep on my bed, and they on theirs. Bad news for cat owners: sleeping with one's cat can be rough, since your sweet kitty's circadian rhythm is quite different from yours[‡] (and perhaps they feel less guilty for loudly demanding your attention at random hours of the night).

---

[*] Henning Johannes Drews, Sebastian Wallot, Philip Brysch, Hannah Berger-Johannsen, Sara Lena Weinhold, Panagiotis Mitkidis, Paul Christian Baier, Julia Lechinger, Andreas Roepstorff, and Robert Göder, "Bed-Sharing in Couples Is Associated with Increased and Stabilized REM Sleep and Sleep-Stage Synchronization," *Frontiers in Psychiatry* 11 (June 2020): 1. https://doi.org/10.3389/FPSYT.2020.00583.

[†] Salma I. Patel, Bernie W. Miller, Heidi E. Kosiorek, James M. Parish, Philip J. Lyng, and Lois E. Krahn, "The Effect of Dogs on Human Sleep in the Home Sleep Environment," *Mayo Clinic Proceedings* 92, no. 9 (2017): 1368–72. https://doi.org/10.1016/J.MAYOCP.2017.06.014.

[‡] Lieve T. van Egmond, Olga E. Titova, Eva Lindberg, Tove Fall, and Christian Benedict, "Association between Pet Ownership and Sleep in the Swedish CArdioPulmonary BioImage Study (SCAPIS)," *Scientific Reports* 11, no. 1 (2017). https://doi.org/10.1038/S41598-021-87080-7.

Going to Bed at the Right Time

In order to cuddle with my partner and dogs, I used to go to bed about an hour before I really wanted to. Because I have a naturally later chronotype, this often meant that I was the last one awake, twiddling my thumbs while listening to multiple snoring bodies around me. Many of my insomnia patients are going to bed too early. They haven't saved up enough sleep drive and their circadian rhythm hasn't reached the right point in the twenty-four-hour cycle. And the most common reason they cite for going to bed before feeling sleepy is that their partner goes to bed early. Sleeping apart could free you to sleep and wake by your natural rhythm.

Better Air Quality

There is clear evidence that air pollution is not good for sleep, whether it's general air pollution in your neighborhood or bad air quality in the bedroom during the night.* Not that I'm comparing my partner's breathing and other bodily functions to air pollution (because he will read this one day), but I must say that when we do share a bed, my sleep is significantly better with the windows open. This makes sense— our bodies and brains function better with plentiful oxygen while we're awake, and there's no reason this would be different while we're asleep. Years ago, when I slept in a small room with a 180-pound human and over two hundred pounds of dogs, I was almost certainly breathing too much carbon dioxide. But, of course, this is an extreme example. If your home is well-ventilated and you only have one other creature in your bedroom, this may not be an issue.

---

* Jianghong Liu, Tina Wu, Qisijing Liu, Shaowei Wu, and Jiu Chiuan Chen, "Air Pollution Exposure and Adverse Sleep Health across the Life Course: A Systematic Review," *Environmental Pollution* 262 (July 2020): 114263. https://doi.org/10.1016/J.ENVPOL.2020.114263.

I Should Sleep Apart from My Partner?
Won't That Be Bad for Our Relationship?

In our culture, a couple sleeping apart is assumed to have a bad relationship. This is silly. When you're both unconscious, there is no reason for you to be on the same surface. It's not like you're having meaningful conversations or making major life decisions together during sleep. In fact, if you're both getting better sleep, it might help your relationship because everyone would be in a better mood.

If you simply love to be in bed together, or you're concerned about decreased sexual intimacy from sleeping apart, you can still get the best of both worlds. My partner and I spend some time snuggling and chatting in bed at his bedtime, then I leave and continue my own evening while he goes to sleep. This way, we still get to go to bed together, but also each enjoy undisturbed, highly oxygenated sleep, each according to our own natural circadian rhythm. This is not to say that you *must* sleep apart from your partner to improve your sleep. For many people, the comfort of bed-sharing is highly beneficial for their overall well-being. If that's the case, by all means, enjoy it! You can decrease the potential sleep disturbances by using earplugs and eye masks, going to bed when you're sleepy, and keeping the bedroom well-ventilated.

BEDROOM BUDDIES CHECKLIST

☐ If dogs are in the bedroom overnight, they are sleeping in their own bed.

☐ Cats are well-provisioned and trained to stay out of the bedroom overnight.

☐ If a human bed partner snores or has obstructive sleep apnea, sleep in separate rooms or use good earplugs.

☐ If you or your bed partner moves a lot or otherwise disturbs the other's sleep, consider sleeping in separate rooms.

☐ If sleeping in separate rooms, consider still going to bed together before lights-out, if this is an enjoyable ritual.

☐ Keep the bedroom well-ventilated by opening the window/door and keeping a fan on.

Screens in the Evening

You've probably heard that bright light in the evening inhibits melatonin and disturbs sleep. Here's the theory behind why that would happen: The brain's master circadian clock, the suprachiasmatic nucleus (SCN), helps us to be sleepy at night and awake during the day, in part by regulating when melatonin is released. Melatonin should ramp up in the evenings and subside in the wee hours of the morning. How does the SCN know when to encourage melatonin release? Light. If there's a lot of light coming in through the eyes, the SCN knows it's daytime. If there's much less light coming in, it must be nighttime. Specifically, short wavelength light (blue light, which is also part of broad spectrum light), tells the SCN that it's daytime and suppresses melatonin release. If we get too much bright light exposure in the evening, such as from electronic devices, we may suppress melatonin release, increase alertness, and interfere with sleep.

Indeed, there's evidence that people who are exposed to more screen light in the evenings have worse sleep, more sluggish mornings, and generally don't feel as good about their sleep.* In the lab, under well-controlled conditions, two hours of short wavelength (blue) light expo-

---

* Michal Šmotek, Eva Fárková, Denisa Manková, and Jana Kopřivová, "Evening and Night Exposure to Screens of Media Devices and Its Association with Subjectively Perceived Sleep: Should 'Light Hygiene' Be given More Attention?" *Sleep Health* 6, no. 4 (2020): 498–505. https://doi.org/10.1016/J.SLEH.2019.11.007.

sure in the late evening not only made sleep more fragmented but also led to more daytime sleepiness and attention issues the next day.* In the real world, sleep researchers got an opportunity to see what would happen when the whole population suddenly started to use their screens even more than usual: during the first weeks of the COVID-19 lockdowns in 2020, Italian researchers surveyed more than two thousand people about their new screen habits and found that those who increased their electronic device use also felt their sleep worsen, including having more insomnia symptoms.†

Studies such as these are not perfect. For example, in the COVID-19 lockdown era study, people who used their devices a lot more might also have experienced other big life changes—unemployment, social isolation, more sedentariness during the day—all things that would also worsen sleep. But still, the growing research on screen use and sleep is interesting enough that I'm taking measures to decrease my blue light exposure, right now, as I type on my laptop at 9:13 P.M. However, before you swear to evening screen celibacy, let's discuss some clarifiers and caveats.

The Amount of Evening Light Exposure Matters Less
Than the Amount of Daytime Light Exposure

Everything is relative. Our brains don't just consider how much evening light there is when regulating melatonin release. They also consider our *recent photic history*, as in how much light exposure we got earlier during

---

* A. Green, M. Cohen-Zion, A. Haim, and Y. Dagan, "Evening Light Exposure to Computer Screens Disrupts Human Sleep, Biological Rhythms, and Attention Abilities," *Chronobiology International* 34, no. 7 (2017): 855–65. https://doi.org/10.1080/07420528.2017.1324878.

† Federico Salfi, Giulia Amicucci, Domenico Corigliano, Aurora D'Atri, Lorenzo Viselli, Daniela Tempesta, and Michele Ferrara, "Changes of Evening Exposure to Electronic Devices during the COVID-19 Lockdown Affect the Time Course of Sleep Disturbances," *Sleep* 44, no. 9 (2021): 1–9, https://doi.org/10.1093/SLEEP/ZSAB080.

the day. In fact, this is so powerful that getting bright light during the day erases the problematic effects of screen use in the evening. For example, Swedish researchers had participants come to their lab in the afternoon, spend about six and a half hours in this brightly lit environment, then read a physical book or an ebook on a tablet for two hours before bedtime. All participants then underwent overnight sleep monitoring. There were absolutely no sleep differences among participants who read a paper book versus those who read an ebook. They had the same sleep quantity, sleep quality, melatonin profile, and next-day functioning.*

This may seem to contradict other studies, which found that two hours of bright evening screen use disturbs sleep, but the difference here is that all participants spent a big chunk of their daytime in bright light. For reference, the brightly lit lab was at about 569 lux, somewhat brighter than a typical office with windows. A typical living room is about 200 lux, a cloudy day 20,000 lux, and direct sun 100,000 lux.

If you work in a somewhat dark environment during the day (e.g., your home office, a cubicle, warehouse, lab), install more broad spectrum lights, sit closer to a window, or best yet, go for an outdoor walk during your lunch break. Get creative and find ways to get daylight exposure. This will go a long way to make your evening screen use a non-problem for sleep.

You Can Easily Mitigate the Effects of Evening Light

Instead of abstaining from screens in the evening entirely, which is not feasible for many of us, you can tone down their impact. Short wavelength lights (e.g., blue) is what suppresses melatonin. Long wavelength

* Frida H. Rångtell, Emelie Ekstrand, Linnea Rapp, Anna Lagermalm, Lisanne Liethof, Marcela Olaya Búcaro, David Lingfors, Jan Erik Broman, Helgi B. Schiöth, and Christian Benedict, "Two Hours of Evening Reading on a Self-Luminous Tablet vs. Reading a Physical Book Does Not Alter Sleep after Daytime Bright Light Exposure," *Sleep Medicine* 23 (July 2016): 111–18. https://doi.org/10.1016/j.sleep.2016.06.016.

lights (e.g., orange) do not. There is not yet perfect consensus among researchers on whether Night Shift mode on smartphones or blue light–blocking glasses really work, but the evidence is leaning toward these being at least somewhat helpful. People are especially likely to benefit from blue light–blocking glasses if they have insomnia, attention-deficit/hyperactivity disorder, bipolar disorder, delayed sleep phase disorder (a.k.a. extreme night owls), or combinations of them.* I have personally found them to be helpful, even though I only have a moderately late chronotype (i.e., not severe enough to be considered a delayed sleep phase disorder).

For example, one study found that wearing blue light–blocking glasses for two hours in the evening made people with insomnia feel significantly better about their sleep, and even increased actual sleep duration by about the same amount that the most popular insomnia medications do (about twenty-eight minutes per night).† Another study combined blue light–blocking glasses with cognitive behavioral therapy for insomnia (CBT-I), and found that the glasses enhanced overall treatment.‡

Although there are still very few studies on this topic, the findings seem promising. You can find blue light–blocking glasses in many stores, including online, for less than twenty dollars. I recommend getting a pair with orange- or amber-colored lenses, because sometimes the clear ones are not great at blocking out short wavelength lights. You can wear them for a couple of hours before bedtime. Do *not* wear them during

* Ari Shechter, Kristal A. Quispe, Jennifer S. Mizhquiri Barbecho, Cody Slater, and Louise Falzon, "Interventions to Reduce Short-Wavelength ('Blue') Light Exposure at Night and Their Effects on Sleep: A Systematic Review and Meta-Analysis," *SLEEP Advances* 1, no. 1 (2020): 1–13. https://doi.org/10.1093/SLEEPADVANCES/ZPAA002.

† Ari Shechter, Elijah Wookhyun Kim, Marie Pierre St-Onge, and Andrew J. Westwood, "Blocking Nocturnal Blue Light for Insomnia: A Randomized Controlled Trial," *Journal of Psychiatric Research* 96 (January 2018): 196–202. https://doi.org/10.1016/J.JPSYCHIRES.2017.10.015.

‡ Karolina Janků, Michal Šmotek, Eva Fárková, and Jana Kopřivová, "Block the Light and Sleep Well: Evening Blue Light Filtration as a Part of Cognitive Behavioral Therapy for Insomnia," *Chronobiology International* 37, no. 2 (2020): 248–59. https://doi.org/10.1080/07420528.2019.1692859.

the day (unless indicated by your eye doctor), because this may backfire and worsen your circadian rhythm. Remember that the *contrast* between light exposure during the day versus night is key to proper melatonin release.

If You Have a Later Chronotype, Your Circadian Rhythm May Be More Sensitive to Evening Light

If you are prone to procrastinating going to bed, like Wei, or you easily slip into a later-to-bed and later-to-rise pattern during vacations, you may have a later chronotype. This means you're biologically hardwired to prefer sleeping and waking later than what is conventional. You may also be more sensitive to the phase-delaying effects of evening bright light. This means your evening screen use, if excessive, could push your sleep timing even later, and that effect is stronger for you than for the average person. That's why, if you know yourself to be a natural night owl, it's worth taking extra care to get lots of bright light during the day, use blue light–blocking glasses in the evening, and give yourself ample screen-free wind-down time before bed (about thirty minutes at least).

The Content on Your Screens (and on Your Mind) Likely Matters More Than the Light Exposure Itself

Not all screens are equal. Reading a Jane Austen novel on a Kindle, for example, is likely not as stimulating as playing a first-person shooter video game. There are no hard-and-fast rules about what content you should or shouldn't consume because what's meaningful or relaxing to one person may not be for another. And there's no need to scrub your evening clean of anything stimulating, because twiddling your thumbs in boredom is not good for your sleep either. That's what happened with

Keisha—she was so lonely and bored in the evenings without any electronic devices that her resulting angst gave her more insomnia than any
screen could have.

What I would recommend is to be honest with yourself about
whether your evening media consumption is fulfilling and enjoyable,
or whether you're just watching TV as a distraction or scrolling social
media for lack of anything else inspiring. **Try to find a balance of intentionally consuming content that adds to your well-being *and* try
to explore nonmedia activities that satisfy your body and mind.** An
example evening could be: Watch your favorite TV show and catch up
with friends on social media, then do a little stretching and journaling.
Cuddle with your dog. Finish up the evening with an episode of light-
hearted Jimmy Kimmel while getting ready for bed, then go to bed with
a book.

MY INTENTIONAL ELECTRONIC DEVICE USE PLAN

It would be enjoyable or meaningful for me to engage in these screen-
related activities in the evening:

☐ Watch these specific TV/streaming shows: _____
(duration _____ minutes)

☐ Engage with these social media platforms:

  ☐ Facebook, for the purpose of _____
  (duration _____ minutes)

  ☐ Twitter, for the purpose of _____
  (duration _____ minutes)

  ☐ Instagram, for the purpose of _____
  (duration _____ minutes)

  ☐ TikTok, for the purpose of _____
  (duration _____ minutes)

☐ Snapchat, for the purpose of _____

(duration _____ minutes)

☐ iMessage or related, for the purpose of _____

(duration _____ minutes)

☐ Other, for the purpose of _____

(duration _____ minutes)

☐ Play these video/phone/tablet games:_____

(duration _____ minutes)

☐ Engage with these websites/forums: _____

(duration _____ minutes)

☐ Engage with these apps: _____

(duration _____ minutes)

☐ Other, for the purpose of: _____

(duration _____ minutes)

It would be enjoyable or meaningful for me to engage in these non-screen activities in the late evenings:

☐ Stretching or light exercise

☐ Reading a book

☐ Journaling

☐ Spending time with partner

☐ Spending time with family, pets

☐ Catching up with friends

☐ Practicing mindfulness or meditation

☐ Engaging in self-pampering: _____

☐ Engaging in a creative process: _____

☐ Doing a hobby: _____

☐ Doing light house chores: _____

☐ Other: _____

☐ Other: _____

I will mitigate the potential problems of evening light exposure by:

☐ Getting lots of bright light exposure during the day

☐ Going outside at these times: _____

☐ Adding broad spectrum light to my indoor work environment
with: _____

☐ Other: _____

☐ Getting less bright light in the evenings

☐ Reducing my screen time to: _____

☐ Wearing blue light–blocking glasses

I have made these changes to help me align with the above plan:

☐ Set reminders on my smartphone to start/stop certain activities (e.g., going outside, checking work email, starting wind-down time)

☐ Enabled my tablet and smartphone's Night Shift mode to automatically turn on in the evening

☐ Made Downtime (iOS) or Focus Mode (Android) settings to limit app notifications in the evening

☐ Enabled time management settings in smartphone/tablet apps so that I'm reminded when I have reached my desired time spent on specific apps

☐ Purchased any necessary light exposure items (e.g., light box for office desk, blue light–blocking glasses)

☐ Rewarded myself for sticking with the plan for a week

Both Keisha and Wei ended up having a much better relationship with sleep and better overall health by the end of insomnia treatment. The biggest change for Keisha was that she no longer analyzed her sleep all the time, which took the pressure off and allowed her to naturally transition to sleepy mode at night. The biggest change for Wei was that he established a more consistent biological schedule, and learned to be more intentional about what activities he wanted to spend time with and when. For example, he still wanted to trade cryptocurrencies, but decided to limit it to fifteen minutes per day in the mornings instead of all day and night, so he put the trading app on the last page of his smartphone screen and disabled notifications to avoid temptation.

Neither of them has perfect sleep hygiene, and that's the point. Keisha needed to move away from perfection, and Wei needed to move toward it. Through some reflection and tinkering, you'll figure out which direction you need to go in too.

BOTTOM LINE

- Exercising in the evening is totally fine.
- Having a TV on during the night (or other significant light/noise in the bedroom) is disruptive to sleep.
- Generally speaking, psychoactive substances (anything that changes your brain's perceptions or functioning) are not great for sleep if used excessively. This includes caffeine, alcohol, nicotine, and recreational drugs. CBD might have short-term benefits for some aspects of sleep, but like any other over-the-counter sleep aid, it's likely not the answer to chronic insomnia.
- However, that doesn't mean you need to or should cut out substances completely for the sake of sleep. Many people have small to moderate amounts of coffee and alcohol, for example, while maintaining a great relationship with sleep. Just know your own sensitivity to these substances, and when in doubt, you can try to reduce your consumption to see if it helps.
- Bed partners (human and animal) can disrupt sleep through their movements, noises, and use of oxygen in the room. They might also make

you go to bed at a time that doesn't suit your chronotype. You can try sleeping separately or using earplugs, eye masks, and better ventilation to mitigate these possible problems.

- Excessive light exposure in the late evening can interfere with sleep and cause next-day fatigue. You may be especially prone to light's interference with your sleep and circadian rhythm if you're already more of a night owl by nature.
- BUT, getting lots of bright light exposure during the day can decrease (or even erase) the problematic effects of screens at night. Go out for a walk if you can.
- Also consider what media you're consuming on your electronic devices at night and why. Find a balance of screen and nonscreen activities that are enjoyable or meaningful to fill your evenings.

12

Looking Back, Planning Ahead

*How to Maintain Your Gains, Get Through Rough Patches,
and Keep a Lifelong Healthy Relationship with Sleep*

S leep often continues to improve in the months after finishing for-
mal treatment for insomnia. According to my ongoing analyses
of dozens of cognitive behavioral therapies for insomnia (CBT-I)
clinical trials, participants are finishing their treatment feeling better
and getting about an *additional* twenty minutes more sleep by three to
twelve months later. This is good news, because whatever gains you've
experienced by guiding yourself through the Hello Sleep program,
they're likely to stick around, and things may get even better.

But of course, every relationship needs to be maintained. In fact, the
more intimate a relationship is, the less we should take it for granted, as
any happily married couple will tell you. Your relationship with sleep is
no different. Now that you've reset your sleep and circadian physiology,
learned skills for shifting your perspective on sleep, and let go of unhelpful sleep effort, you've earned a healthier relationship with your oldest
friend.

Now it's time to review the major concepts and skills you used to get here and those you want to continue working on. And let's not wait until something goes wrong to act. Let's start with how we can take initiative that will keep the relationship solid in the long term.

Be Appreciative

One of my recent patients, Wayne, was, by the numbers, an all-star. He used to take an average of two hours to fall asleep, but by the end of treatment he was only taking an average of thirty minutes. He had even reduced his sleep medication use by about 75 percent, and was on track to completely quit. I was so excited to review his progress with him during his last session. To my surprise, he was still quite unsatisfied with his sleep. It turned out that he was still concerned about waking up (briefly) one to two times per night. He was disappointed that after all his hard work, he was still not able to "sleep through the night."

Wayne's experience is not uncommon. Sometimes we become so focused on the goal of improving sleep that we can only see what is yet imperfect. And sometimes that last fly in the ointment can loom frustratingly large.

Even aside from the fact that waking up a couple of times per night is totally normal and healthy, Wayne was forgetting to see the big picture. When we zoomed out and reviewed all the ways in which his sleep (and his relationship with sleep) had changed, he suddenly saw just how far he had come in a few weeks. He said, "Wow, if you had described my current sleep pattern to my past self from three months ago, I would have thought it was a pipe dream!" Indeed, Wayne became more and more amazed at how much was going well with his sleep, and how much his imperfect, yet wonderful, sleep was doing for his overall quality of life. Let's do the same as Wayne and start our happily-ever-after with sleep by appreciating it. Ask yourself,

- What do I appreciate about sleep? How does sleep help me?
- How have things changed for the better with sleep?
- What is going well with sleep? What is going well with my overall well-being?

To help yourself answer these questions, compare your sleep log data from before you started the Hello Sleep program to your data from the most recent week. If you're using the Consensus Sleep Diary app, look at the graphs that show your changes over the past several weeks. What's changed in this data? What about things that these numbers don't capture, like the amount of time you spend ruminating about sleep? Also give yourself credit for prioritizing and investing in your relationship with sleep. Ask yourself,

- What skills and knowledge do I have now that I didn't before?
- What am I doing well to support my relationship with sleep?
- What do I feel more confident about now?
- What unhelpful patterns have I overcome?

Take your time to feel proud and appreciative. This isn't just for the sake of warm and fuzzy feelings (although this is reason enough!). Being able to appreciate your sleep, now and anytime in the future, is a crucial skill for weathering temporary setbacks and changes in your sleep pattern.

WRITE A LOVE LETTER TO YOUR SLEEP

This is a cheesy (and optional) exercise that I personally love. Simply write a love letter to your sleep as if it were a person. Literally start with, "Dear Sleep . . ." and list all the ways in which you love and appreciate it. Pretend you're a 1990s boy band singer (or Adele, or a Beatle), walking with sleep on a romantic beach, tortured with infatuation. Make promises about what you'll do to show your love. Keep this letter for future review during rough patches.

Be Giving and Supportive

One major red flag for any toxic relationship is when one party is always taking, taking, taking, demanding, demanding, demanding. Expecting a partner to perform and provide, without putting equal investment into the partnership, is a sure way to sabotage a relationship. If you find yourself becoming frustrated that your sleep sucks, that it's not giving you what you need, let's pause and see if you're giving sleep what it needs from you. After all, your body and brain are not miracle workers and can only work with what you give them. Here are good places to start:

- Continue light + movement routine, which includes,
  - » getting lots of light exposure during the day, especially in the morning;*
  - » minimizing bright light exposure in the late evenings by dimming screens or wearing blue light–blocking glasses;† and
  - » being physically active, even if briefly, every day. It doesn't have to be intense exercise, just consistent and often.

----

* Quick refresher: This should include being outside whenever possible, and if you must spend long hours indoors, broad spectrum light from a light box for thirty minutes in the morning. No matter how much light you have in your indoor office, add more, especially if you're not sitting directly in front of a large window.

† Remember, the point isn't to avoid light exposure in general, it's to have a big contrast between how much light you get during the day versus at night. There is no need to cut out screens overall in the evenings.

- Keeping consistent life rhythms, which include,
  - » getting up at about the same time every day, including days off; and
  - » eating regular meals at about the same time every day— don't skip breakfast.
- Being intentional and reasonable with substances.* When in doubt,
  - » try reducing caffeine intake;
  - » try reducing alcohol intake;
  - » try reducing or quitting nicotine;
  - » reduce or eliminate other psychoactive drugs (including cannabis); and
  - » review your sleep medications (and other medications that may affect sleep) with your doctor.
- Creating a welcoming environment for sleep (without going overboard with perfectionism):
  - » Make sure your sleeping environment is well ventilated.
  - » Wear earplugs or an eye mask if there's excessive noise/ light in your sleep environment.
  - » Consider sleeping apart from your partner (or pets) if either of you snores or moves a lot.
- Investing in general healthy habits, such as having good nutrition and addressing health problems promptly when they arise.

Be a Good Listener

One of the most amazing things about sleep is that it adapts to your needs. Whether you're training for a marathon or recovering from ill-

---

* When reducing/quitting substances, be patient, because the withdrawal symptoms will likely make sleep feel worse before it starts to get better. I highly recommend working with a behavioral healthcare provider when you're working on a difficult quit (e.g., cigarettes).

ness or having a particularly emotional experience, your body will automatically adjust sleep to support the most important endeavor of the moment. Your body listens to you. But we often don't listen to our bodies. Instead, we hold expectations and make demands of our bodies, getting frustrated when they don't perform as we want them to. In a one-way relationship like this, we drift further and further away from knowing what our bodies need, and we impose our own arbitrary ideas of how sleep *should* be, straining our relationship with it. Here's how we can be a good listener:

- **Approach your body with mindful curiosity.** Regularly practice mindful breathing and body scans, even if very briefly. Remember that "mindful" simply means being in the here-and-now without judging anything as good or bad. Simply notice what your body feels.

- **Remember that sleepy and tired are totally different things.** When you feel like you just want to curl up in bed, ask yourself which of these you feel. If you feel sleepy, it's time to go to bed.* If you feel tired (or run down, worn out, exhausted, bored, sluggish, etc.), ask your body what it really needs.

- **Don't automatically use caffeine (or other substances) to overcome fatigue.** You don't have to quit coffee. Have it because you enjoy it, or because you like the jolt that one cup in the morning gives you, not because you need multiple jolts to keep your day going. If you feel like you can't function without caffeine, ask your body what it really needs.

- **Pain is not "weakness leaving your body." It's a cry for help.** Don't push through pain and other alarm signals, like signs of

---

* And if you often feel sleepy during the day, outside of a regularly timed brief nap, it's time to consult a doctor about possible sleep apnea or to review your medications.

burnout. Resting and nurturing your body is not weak or self-indulgent. It's the responsible thing to do.

- **Don't think of sleep as a performance enhancer.** To the tech enthusiasts trying to top the scoreboard on their sleep tracking apps, sleeping 5 percent more doesn't mean you increase your performance by 5 percent. Seeing your sleep as a means to greater productivity alienates you from what really matters—a curiosity for what your body really needs for true well-being.
- **Always be open to change.** There is beauty and wonder in change. Your sleep may be different from week to week, season to season, and certainly, year to year. Don't hold tightly to expectations based on how things used to be. Be curious about what your body needs now, which might be less or more sleep than before, or sleep in a different pattern. The only "right" way in any given moment is what satisfies your body.

Have Realistic and Fair Expectations

Another common thing that trips up people's long-term relationship with sleep is the "expectation creep." You tell yourself, "Yes, things are much better, but I still sometimes have rough nights: Shouldn't I be able to sleep well every night? I do feel better during the day, but I'm still sluggish for a while every morning. Shouldn't I be able to jump out of bed, ready to go? Okay, now I don't really have insomnia anymore, but I really want to sleep 5 percent more so I can perform 5 percent better."

Remember, you're a human . . . not a robot. So many factors affect our sleep, mood, energy levels, and even our perception of these things, that we can't possibly control all of them. Even if we could, we'd be spending our life preventing imperfections rather than truly living. Here are some quick reminders about what is totally normal to have in a healthy relationship with sleep:

- **You *should* be waking up a handful of times per night.** It's okay if you don't remember most or any of these awakenings. Even if you do remember a few, that's perfectly normal and does not indicate poor sleep quality.

- **Everyone has insomnia sometimes.** I certainly do! This doesn't mean your overall sleep health or relationship with sleep is bad.

- **Most people wake up feeling groggy, unmotivated, sluggish.** This is called "sleep inertia" and is completely normal. It takes about half an hour of moving the body for our system to boot up.

- **Sometimes you'll sleep well and still be tired during the day.** That's because most things that cause fatigue are not sleep related. Remember to hydrate, eat well, move, socialize, rest, reflect, feed your creativity, and accept that being tired sometimes (or even often, if you're a parent) is a normal part of the human condition.

- **Some people will always have an easier time with falling/ staying asleep than you.** This does not mean that your sleep is bad, or even that their sleep is better than yours. In fact, if you have people in your life that can fall asleep at the drop of a hat and are able to snore away under any condition . . . they may want to be screened for sleep apnea. That's because falling asleep this easily indicates excessive sleepiness, a common sign of a sleep disorder.

- **You don't need to have a perfect "sleep score."** Your sleep tracker, if you ever decide to use one again, may not be accurate in reporting your sleep, especially when it comes to sleep stages. The sleep scores they give you may also be close to meaningless, depending on how they're calculated. It's better to trust your relationship with sleep and rely on the contextualized knowledge you now have about your sleep.

Be Flexible and Forgiving Instead of Overbearing

Even with generally realistic and fair expectations, it can be frustrating when things change, sometimes inexplicably. In human relationships, sometimes your friend cancels a dinner date last-minute, or your partner is grumpy for seemingly no reason. We can choose to fixate on the event, trying to play detective about why it happened and ruminating about how it shouldn't be like this, or we can accept that sometimes things aren't perfect, and we'll never know why and that's okay. If we are flexible and forgiving with occasional sleep problems, we will have a much easier time maintaining an overall good relationship with sleep. This is especially true for people who are prone to insomnia because insomnia positively *feeds* on rumination, overanalyzing, and rigid expectations. Remember sleep effort? Here's a refresher on how to let go of it:

- **Let perfectionism be a red flag.** If you find yourself thinking, "If only this *one* thing about sleep was just a *little* bit better . . ." or "But if I could just go that last half mile to achieve X . . .", take a step back and reflect on what's already going well. Be patient. Stick with what you *can* control and let go of what you haven't been able to.
- **Stop doing research about how to improve your sleep.** The vast majority of online articles about sleep have incomplete, misleading, or downright incorrect content, and they'll just shake your confidence and trap you in the quicksand of sleep effort. Also, thank your family and friends for their concern, but ask them to please stop sending you articles about sleep.
- **Don't plan your life around sleep.** Keep a generally consistent set of life rhythms, as discussed above, but don't turn down social or travel opportunities just because they'll temporarily disrupt your sleep schedule. If you're having fun at a party or want

to indulge in that extra cocktail, don't let perfect sleep hygiene be the reason to stop you.

- **Don't spend a lot of money on sleep.** If you want to indulge in a premium mattress simply because it feels good for your back, go for it! But if you find yourself considering spending big dollars specifically to "level up" your sleep or to prevent insomnia, know that you don't need to. All you're buying is sleep effort and unreasonable expectations.

- **Let go of sleep tracking gadgets.** I must sound like a broken record about this but I can't help but wonder how much angst about sleep would evaporate if people with insomnia (or past insomnia) simply dropped this habit. Trust yourself and your sleep. Tracking sleep with a gadget that doesn't even give you actionable and clinically sound advice is just being overbearing.

- **Most important, don't *try* to make yourself fall asleep.** Whether it's through meditation, counting sheep, turning on or off gadgets, if you're doing something specifically to induce sleep, you're trying too hard. If sleep doesn't want to come to you right now, no amount of persuasion will change that. Attempts to persuade it will only push sleep even farther away. Get out of bed and do something enjoyable with your extra "me" time.

How to Reset When You Hit a Rough Patch

Inevitably, we will go through periods of stress, travel, schedule disruption, health changes, and other events that can throw us off track with sleep. Over the course of a lifetime, your sleep needs and patterns will also change. Menopause, for example, is notorious for shaking up sleep patterns. Insomnia relapse sometimes happens. It's not particularly common for people who have gone through treatments similar to the

Hello Sleep program, but if it does happen, know that it's a normal feature in a lifelong relationship with sleep.

If you find yourself in the thick of insomnia again, don't panic and don't beat yourself up. You'll already be in a better place than before you read this book by virtue of having knowledge and experience with overcoming insomnia. You'll also have a solid foundation with sleep by being appreciative, giving sleep what it needs, keeping fair expectations, and being flexible.

Against this backdrop, there are some concrete things you can do in response to sleep changes.

When You're in the Thick of a Sleep-Disrupting Event, Just Listen to Your Body: Don't Hold Too Tightly to Rules

The bamboo that bends in the wind doesn't break. We have to be flexible when circumstances change, which means listening to what your body needs instead of sticking with rules. For example, if you've just had surgery, don't try to precisely keep to your previous sleep-wake schedule. Just sleep and rest as much as your body wants to while doing your best to still get bright light exposure during the day. If you've just had a baby and you're providing nighttime care, take as many naps as you need during the day while you work on inching your newborn toward having a day versus night pattern.* If you're experiencing an extraordinarily stressful (but probably temporary) circumstance—let's say you're getting a divorce and in the process of moving out—and you just don't have the wherewithal to practice ideal stress management for these few weeks, know that sleep medications were invented for exactly

---

* Babies are not born with clear day versus night circadian rhythms in their sleep pattern. Don't worry. They develop it within the first three months of life, after which they'll sleep much more at night than during the day. You can help by giving them light exposure during the day and keeping lights dim at night.

this type of situation. There's nothing wrong with taking them (when prescribed by your doctor, of course) to get relief before you get to reset your relationship with sleep.

Because the array of circumstances you might encounter is so diverse, there's no way for me to give you specific direction about how exactly to roll with the punches. When in doubt, listen to your body. If you're sleepy, that means you need sleep. If you're not sleepy even when you desperately want to sleep, that means you need something else, such as emotional support from your partner or a warm bath, and you shouldn't try to force sleep. Still try your best to stick to consistent rhythms, bright light exposure during the day, and other generally good physical and mental health habits. When your stressful circumstance calms down or you settle into a coping state, you can move on to the next steps.

When You're Ready to Focus on Sleep Health Again, Start with Keeping Sleep Logs

Often, simply the act of keeping daily sleep logs for a week or two will improve things. You'll get a bird's-eye view of what your sleep-wake patterns are and be reminded of things that helped you the first time you went through the Hello Sleep program. For example, you might notice that you're spending a lot more time in bed than you realized, or that your wake-up times vary dramatically across the week. You may even see that things are different from the last time you had chronic insomnia, and you need to focus on different skills this time.

Do the Big Reset Again, if Needed

If you find yourself well into an insomnia pattern again, with frequent difficulty with falling/staying asleep, letting go of the racing mind, or generally feeling like your sleep pattern is unpredictable and unsatisfying, it might be time to turn back to part II of this book (The Big Reset). Depending on what your sleep logs show, you may need to steady your sleep-wake timing, shorten your time spent in bed, or start consistently getting out of bed when you're struggling to fall asleep (or falling back to sleep). You may find that this reset is easier the second time around because you're likely starting from a better place and already know what to expect.

Pay Attention to the Way You're Thinking and Feeling About Sleep

It's easy to fall back into old ways of thinking. Well-practiced anxieties are difficult to dismantle but easy to pick up again. If you find yourself ruminating about sleep, blaming sleep for your problems, getting frustrated with sleeplessness during the night, or generally having lots of angst about sleep, it's time to revisit part III of this book (Going Deeper into the Relationship). You may want to keep track of your sleep-related thoughts (they're often harder to identify than you'd think!) for a week and refresh your pocket Socrates skills. The sleep effort chapter (chapter 9) may also be a good reminder of what behaviors are not so helpful, even if they really seem like they should be. And don't forget—you've overcome insomnia before. Trust yourself to do it again, and trust in your relationship with sleep.

Consult a Sleep Specialist, if Needed

Instead of piecing together dubious information from the internet, invest in a consultation, if possible, with a behavioral sleep medicine specialist. We are knowledgeable about not only the science of sleep, but the clinical practice of understanding your sleep in the context of your whole person and providing guidance accordingly. If you've already gone through the Hello Sleep program, you'll likely need less one-on-one time with a specialist. Most of us provide services that are at least partially covered by insurance, so it may be more affordable than you think. My go-to directories for finding a specialist* are:

- The Society of Behavioral Sleep Medicine (behavioralsleep.org /index.php/directory)
- The Penn International CBT-I Directory (cbti.directory)

How to Enjoy the Benefits of a Better Relationship with Sleep

Up to this point, we've covered the ways to improve your relationship with sleep. Let's not forget that the whole point of this is, presumably, to have an overall healthier and more fulfilled life. Sometimes we can get so caught up in solving problems or chasing goals that we forget the "why," so let's close our Hello Sleep journey together by reflecting on how to actually enjoy the benefits of better sleep in a broader sense.

A Better Relationship with Sleep Means More Freedom

Even though we started the Big Reset with some formulaic "rules," that was never the ultimate goal. The whole point of starting fresh and reimagining our relationship with sleep is to gain more freedom in your life, instead of being shackled by rules, guilt, anxieties, and other things that come with insomnia. By now, you are hopefully not having to closely monitor your sleep-wake timing (yes, you can stop doing sleep

---

* Note that providers with "DBSM" or "CBSM" after their names are generally those with the highest level of expertise in this specialty area. These credentials mean that they are certified by the Board of Behavioral Sleep Medicine or the American Board of Sleep Medicine.

logs now!) or sleep-related thoughts. If you are still working on these skills, no problem! Go at your own pace, knowing that the ultimate reward is being able to organically respond to changing sleep needs, say "yes" to fun opportunities that will throw sleep off track, and not worry about having perfect sleep hygiene. If you generally maintain a good relationship with sleep, sleep itself no longer feels like work.

More Satisfying Sleep Means Better Mental and Physical Health

Insomnia is a stressor. When we come out of it, we have less mental and physical burden, which translates to less depression and anxiety, less inflammation, less pain, and better coping with other health problems. This might also come with lower healthcare costs, since we know that people with insomnia are usually saddled with higher out-of-pocket medical expenses even if they're not spending directly on insomnia treatment.* Give yourself a pat on the back and maybe buy yourself something nice as a treat.

Better Sleep Means More Bandwidth to Enjoy Life

What do you want to do with the better health and extra time you now have because you are no longer *working* on sleep? Consider if there are any relationships or activities you put on pause (or never started) because you felt too overwhelmed by sleep problems. Even if things are not yet perfect, is it time to

- reconnect with an old friend;
- go out and date more;

---

* Ronald J. Ozminkowski, Shaohung Wang, and James K. Walsh, "The Direct and Indirect Costs of Untreated Insomnia in Adults in the United States," *Sleep* 30, no. 3 (2007): 263–73. https://doi.org/10.1093/SLEEP/30.3.263.

- pick up a new hobby;
- get back to a sport or exercise;
- read fiction (instead of self-help) books;
- have a difficult but necessary conversation;
- reassess your job / career;
- create something; or
- treat yourself.
- Other: _____

More Confidence About Sleep Means You Can
Look at the Bigger Picture

In addition to good sleep health, what else do you value in life? Now that you don't have to pay so much attention to sleep, you can look at the bigger picture of what's important to you. If you haven't considered this recently, or have felt like you've been moving through life on autopilot, it's time to do the old "write your own eulogy" thought experiment. Don't worry, it's not as morbid as it sounds. Simply ask yourself what parts of your life are important to you. What would you like remembered about yourself and your life when it's over? Be honest with yourself. To help you start brainstorming, here are some sample values:

Compassion	Wealth	Mastery	Intimacy	Power
Legacy	Creativity	Independence	Curiosity	Beauty
Health	Community	Justice	Adventure	Contribution
Wisdom	Loyalty	Status	Growth	Family

None of them are mandatory values, nor better or worse than the others. Highlight the ones that speak to you, cross out the ones that don't, and brainstorm more of your own. Sleep on it. Revise your list. Take a small action or two toward an important value that you've been neglecting.

Be patient. Identifying your values and following through on them is a lifelong pursuit, and now that you have a solid relationship with sleep, you have even more freedom to explore.

Wayne took up traveling again. This is something he just didn't feel like he had the wherewithal to do for many years, but now that he wasn't worried about sleep anymore, he started to feel a hankering for adventure. He booked a trip to Germany for Oktoberfest, something he had always wanted to experience. He later told me he didn't sleep much when he was there because he was having so much fun, but that it hadn't bothered him because he trusted his relationship with sleep to be resilient even after jet lag and partying. How refreshing! Now, what would you like to do with this newfound confidence?

BOTTOM LINE

- Congratulations on completing the Hello Sleep program! I hope you are feeling much better in your relationship with sleep.
- To maintain your gains in the long term, you should
  » appreciate sleep and your sleep improvements;
  » give sleep what it needs—consistent rhythms, a welcoming environment, and not too many substances;
  » listen to what your body needs instead of imposing your expectations;
  » have fair and realistic expectations for sleep; and
  » be flexible instead of perfectionistic.
- If you're going through a rough patch with sleep,
  » sleep according to your need (instead of based on rules) when you're in the middle of a sleep-disrupting circumstance;
  » when you're ready to get back on track, start by keeping sleep logs;
  » do the Big Reset (part II of this book) again, if needed;

- » pay attention to how you feel and think about sleep (part III of this book); and
- » consult a sleep specialist, if needed.
- Don't forget to enjoy the fruits of your labor. With a better relationship with sleep, you now have
  - » more freedom in your life from sleep-related rules, anxiety, and guilt;
  - » better health and lower medical costs;
  - » more bandwidth to enjoy life; and
  - » an opportunity to look at the bigger picture of what you value in life.

PART IV

Changes and Challenges in Your Relationship with Sleep

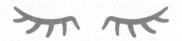

13

Hello Hormones!

Sleep During Pregnancy, Postpartum, and Menopause

As I write these words, my soon-to-be-born baby girl is enthusiastically kicking my bladder. I'm feeling drowsy even though I slept ten hours last night, but I know that I'm going to have trouble falling and staying asleep tonight, which I've been experiencing for the past few weeks. I'm not alone. Seventy-eight percent of people who have been pregnant say the worst sleep of their life was during pregnancy.*

It's wild to me that women's† sleep health does not get a bigger spotlight considering that women are one and a half times more likely to have

---

* Christine H. J. Won, "Sleeping for Two: The Great Paradox of Sleep in Pregnancy," *Journal of Clinical Sleep Medicine* 11, no. 6 (2015): 593–94. https://doi.org/10.5664/JCSM.4760.

† In this chapter, when I say "women" and "mothers," I will be echoing the language used in the research studies I cite. To be honest, I don't know what exactly these terms mean in the research literature. Currently, there is very little research on the sleep of transgender people, and what does exist is mostly about the effect of gender minority stress on sleep. Further, most research on sleep does not distinguish between gender and sex. That's why it's hard to say whether the current knowledge about women's sleep applies to cisgender women only, or everyone with female reproductive organs, or everyone experiencing a specific hormonal or life event (e.g., menopause, becoming a parent), or some other definition. I'll try my best to be precise, and we'll all hope that future research sheds more light on these questions.

insomnia than men.* This difference begins to emerge as early as puberty† and is then exacerbated again during every major reproductive system upheaval (pregnancy, postpartum, menopause). You would think health advocates would be shouting from the rooftops about women's sleep. This topic deserves its own book (or series of books), so this chapter will not do it justice. But I will try my best to summarize the most useful points to know during these rocky times in your relationship with sleep.

How Does Sleep Change During Pregnancy?

Three-quarters of pregnant people report having poor quality sleep, and about half have significant sleep problems. About 38 percent have clinically significant insomnia (almost four times the rate for the general adult population), and it may be even higher for some in their third trimester.‡ This is not surprising, given that pregnancy is a time of dramatic change in every aspect of a person's physical, mental, and social being. Some common sleep-related disturbances by trimester include:§

First Trimester

- Increased daytime sleepiness
- Increased total sleep duration

---

* Sooyeon Suh, Nayoung Cho, and Jihui Zhang, "Sex Differences in Insomnia: From Epidemiology and Etiology to Intervention," *Current Psychiatry Reports* 20, no. 9 (2018): 1–12. https://doi.org/10.1007/S11920-018-0940-9.

† Jihui Zhang, Ngan Yin Chan, Siu Ping Lam, Shirley Xin Li, Yaping Liu, Joey W.Y. Chan, Alice Pik Shan Kong, et al., "Emergence of Sex Differences in Insomnia Symptoms in Adolescents: A Large-Scale School-Based Study." *Sleep* 39, no. 8 (2016): 1563–70. https://doi.org/10.5665/SLEEP.6022.

‡ Ivan D. Sedov, Emily E. Cameron, Sheri Madigan, and Lianne M. Tomfohr-Madsen, "Sleep Quality During Pregnancy: A Meta-Analysis," *Sleep Medicine Reviews* 38 (April 2018): 168–176.

§ Bilgay Izci Balserak, and Kathryn Aldrich Lee, "Sleep and Sleep Disorders Associated with Pregnancy," in *Principles and Practice of Sleep Medicine*, ed. Meir Kryger, Thomas Roth, and William C. Dement (New York: Elsevier, 2017), 1525–39.

- Increased number of nighttime awakenings
- Decreased deep sleep
- Nighttime discomfort (e.g., breast pain, frequent urination)

Second Trimester

- Improved nighttime sleep compared to first trimester
- Less fatigue and daytime sleepiness compared to first trimester
- Onset or worsening of snoring, nasal congestion
- Vivid dreams
- Possible onset of restless legs syndrome
- Back and joint pain

Third Trimester

- Return of fatigue and daytime sleepiness
- Return of fragmented nighttime sleep (i.e., many awakenings)
- Decrease in deep sleep and REM sleep
- Worsening positional discomfort in bed
- Worsening back, joint, and pelvic pain
- Vivid dreams and nightmares
- Increasing risk of obstructive sleep apnea
- Increasing risk of restless legs syndrome

We may not have control over all these sleep changes, but I find that it's helpful to understand why they happen. These clues can help us learn how to cope in the moment and how to return to good sleep after pregnancy.

Hormonal Changes

During the first trimester of pregnancy, human chorionic gonadotropin (HCG) levels approximately double every two days. Progesterone and estrogen also rise dramatically over the course of pregnancy. This mind-boggling amount of hormonal change has direct effects on sleep:

- HCG and progesterone have soporific effects, which is why pregnant people tend to experience a lot more sleepiness during the day and may need to sleep longer at night.
- Progesterone, in a cruel twist, also causes nighttime sleep frag-mentation (i.e., more awakenings). This is part of the reason why pregnant people wake up more often during the night and don't feel as rested even after long nights of sleep.
- Estrogen decreases REM sleep. It can also cause upper airway congestion that induces or worsens snoring and obstructive sleep apnea.
- Hormonal changes also cause other physical symptoms that make sleep more difficult, such as nausea, heartburn, joint dis-comfort, breast pain, and frequent urination.

Anatomical and Physical Changes

Pregnancy can feel like an alien has taken over your body. Sometimes, it is not very kind to your sleep. You may experience:

- rapid pregnancy-related weight gain that can induce or exacer-bate snoring and obstructive sleep apnea;
- abdominal and pelvic pressure that causes discomfort and pain, making it increasingly difficult to find a comfortable position at night;
- nasal congestion, which causes dry mouth, leading to drinking more water at night, and needing to urinate even more often;
- intense fetal movement at night, the baby's favorite time to prac-tice karate in the uterus; and

- for many, worsening iron deficiency that dramatically increases risk for restless legs syndrome, which occurs primarily in the evenings.

Psychological and Emotional Changes

It isn't just the body that undergoes a transformation. During pregnancy, you may experience emotional upheavals and psychological changes that include

- anxiety and depressive symptoms, which are common during pregnancy and can certainly disrupt sleep; and
- "nesting" symptoms, which involves an intense drive to get ready for the baby, which can keep your mind spinning even late into the night.

How to Cope with Sleep Changes During Pregnancy

Sadly, there's not much we can do to prevent most of these pregnancy factors that affect sleep, especially hormonal shifts and physical changes. But it's reassuring to keep in mind that most will not last forever, and that for most people, sleep goes back to normal after pregnancy and the postpartum months. While you're in the midst of it, here are some things you can do to cope:

- **Use the same Hello Sleep approaches, but be more lenient with yourself with the Big Reset portion.** Remember, pregnancy insomnia is short term (even when it feels like forever), and your only job right now is to grow a human and take care of yourself the best that you can. You can try to cope with sleep problems and prevent them from becoming chronic, but don't work so hard that it becomes more stressful than helpful. For example, I wouldn't restrict the time-in-bed window to less than seven hours, or even eight hours if you're usually a longer sleeper. Spending more time resting in bed is fine, as long as you're not experiencing a lot of angst trying to force sleep.

- **During the peaks of excessive sleepiness (first and third trimesters), plan to nap.** Instead of letting yourself doze off during evening TV, which may negatively impact nighttime sleep, set aside an hour (or even two, if possible) to nap or at least rest in the middle of the day. If you're at work and can't nap properly, still try your best to rest during your lunch break instead of eating while working or socializing with coworkers.

- **Keep your wake-up time consistent from day to day, but listen to your body's changing needs.** Consistency is your circadian system's best friend, so don't let your rise time swing wildly throughout the week. But over the course of your pregnancy, allow your sleep schedule to change depending on the current trimester's needs (e.g., after an energetic second trimester you may need to allow a later rise time to get more sleep in the third trimester).

- **Make sure to get plenty of bright light exposure during the day.** This has the double benefit of helping your circadian system *and* setting up your baby for an easier time establishing a day versus night rhythm after they're born. It's not clear exactly how you confer this benefit upon the fetus, but it's certainly a worthwhile investment because trust me, the sooner your baby knows the difference between day and night, the less everyone will cry.

- **Take snoring and signs of obstructive sleep apnea seriously.** If prior to pregnancy you snored or had sleep apnea, it is now more important than ever to treat it, for your health as well as your baby's. If you never snored before, but started during pregnancy, your risk of gestational hypertension and depression are even higher than if you've always snored. Other signs of obstructive sleep apnea include gasping/choking/snorting during sleep, waking up with a headache or dry mouth, and having high blood pressure. Risk factors include being overweight and having a larger collar size (but I've also worked with slim people and top athletes who have apnea, so err on the side of being cautious!). Ask for a referral to a sleep specialist as early as possible, because scheduling testing and receiving treatment can take many weeks.

- **Apply skills from parts II and III of this book to other aspects of life.** For example, you can become more aware of your unhelpful automatic thoughts and walk through your pocket Socrates questions for non-sleep problems. And now is a great time to practice mindfulness even more. These skills can help to alleviate pregnancy-related anxiety, racing mind, and physical stress.
- **Keep up a nutritious diet and consult with a dietician specializing in pregnancy.** This is important overall, but may also help to prevent restless legs syndrome, which is often due to low ferritin levels (i.e., iron stores). A good diet may also help with fatigue.
- **Work with a prenatal physical therapist before you think you need one.** This was the best thing I did for my second pregnancy. There are things you don't know that you don't know, and proper guidance about exercises and posture can help to alleviate pain, prevent injury, and even promote mental health.
- **Establish a relationship with a mental health therapist before you need one.** Better emotional coping means better sleep, and better sleep means better emotional coping. Perinatal depression and anxiety disorders are so common that I think every pregnant person should get some preemptive therapy. This is

especially a good idea if you have a history of mood disorder symptoms, anticipate a difficult delivery, have little social support, or have a history of sleep problems.

How Does Sleep Change Postpartum?

When someone's pregnant, the first thing well-meaning family members (and strangers) say is, "Congratulations!" The second is, "Enjoy your sleep now, because you'll never sleep again once the baby is here." This worried me quite a bit when I was pregnant the first time. My sleep was already awful due to discomfort, hormones, and having to pee every twenty-six minutes . . . and it was going to get *worse*? My concern was warranted because postpartum sleep is undoubtedly important for many aspects of parents' and babies' well-being. For example, researchers have known for decades that postpartum depression is, in part, correlated with infant temperament (e.g., how much a baby cries),* but more recent research finds that if we statistically take the mother's sleep fragmentation into consideration, the temperament-depression relationship disappears.† In other words, it's not really how much the baby cries that matters, but how poorly the mother sleeps that influences her perception of, and reaction to, the baby's temperament, which, in turn, contributes to her mood.

Ironically, the worry about postpartum sleep sometimes kept me up during pregnancy. Since then, I've gained a more nuanced understanding of the research on this topic and some valuable personal experi-

---

* Cheryl Tatano Beck, "A Meta-Analysis of the Relationship between Postpartum Depression and Infant Temperament," *Nursing Research* 45, no. 4 (1996): 225–30. https://doi.org/10.1097/00006199-199607000-00006.

† Deepika Goyal, Caryl Gay, and Kathryn Lee, "Fragmented Maternal Sleep Is More Strongly Correlated with Depressive Symptoms than Infant Temperament at Three Months Postpartum," *Archives of Women's Mental Health* 12, no. 4 (2009): 229–37. https://doi.org/10.1007/S00737-009-0070-9/TABLES/4.

ence (as well as the vicarious experience of my army of mom friends). Here's what you can generally expect with sleep postpartum:

Bad News

- The first one to three months postpartum will be rough for sleep, especially for first-time parents, and especially for those who already had sleep problems.*
- The most obvious sleep disruption is more awakenings at night to feed the baby. There's no getting around this, unless you can regularly afford an overnight postpartum doula, or your partner is able to handle 100 percent of nighttime baby care.
- The less discussed but perhaps bigger problem is profound circadian disruption: mothers tend to experience a dramatic decrease in daytime light exposure from pregnancy to postpartum,† which flattens the melatonin circadian curve and disrupts both nighttime sleep and daytime functioning.
- Another circadian problem: the primary caregiver (and often other caregivers too) sleep less at night and more during the day, which also flattens the day versus night curve for our biological rhythms.‡
- You may also experience other unusual sleep symptoms post-partum due to temporary sleep deprivation, sleep fragmentation, and circadian disruption. They may include:

---

* Lisa M. Christian, Judith E. Carroll, Douglas M. Teti, and Martica H. Hall, "Maternal Sleep in Pregnancy and Postpartum Part I: Mental, Physical, and Interpersonal Consequences," *Current Psychiatry Reports* 21, no. 3 (2019): 1–8. https://doi.org/10.1007/S11920-019-0999-Y.

† Kari Grethe Hjorthaug Gallaher, Anastasiya Slyepchenko, Benicio N. Frey, Kristin Urstad, and Signe K Dørheim, "The Role of Circadian Rhythms in Postpartum Sleep and Mood," *Sleep Medicine Clinics* 13, no. 3 (2018): 359–74. https://doi.org/10.1016/j.jsmc.2018.04.006.

‡ Karen A. Thomas, and Robert L. Burr, "Melatonin Level and Pattern in Postpartum Versus Nonpregnant Nulliparous Women," *Journal of Obstetric, Gynecologic & Neonatal Nursing* 35, no. 5 (2006): 608–15. https://doi.org/10.1111/J.1552-6909.2006.00082.X.

» Nightmares

» Sleep terrors (suddenly waking with intense fear or distress without having had a dream)

» Sleep paralysis (waking up but not being able to move for several seconds or minutes)

» Sleep hallucinations (seeing or hearing things that aren't there as you're falling asleep or waking up)

» Confusional arousals (waking up very disoriented and confused)

Good News

• The baby develops their own circadian rhythm sometime between one and three months of age, which helps everybody get longer stretches of sleep at night.

• Primary caregivers can help babies establish their circadian rhythms by keeping their own rhythms robust* (e.g., more light and activity during the day, less of both at night).

• Parents usually recover normal nighttime sleep efficiency by three months postpartum. If this is your second (or subsequent) baby, your nighttime sleep recovers even more quickly.[†] I personally believe this is because your firstborn forces you to maintain a somewhat normal day versus night rhythm, with plenty of daytime light exposure, because you're wran-

---

* Shao Yu Tsai, Kathryn E. Barnard, Martha J. Lentz, and Karen A. Thomas, "Mother-Infant Activity Synchrony as a Correlate of the Emergence of Circadian Rhythm," *Biological Research for Nursing* 13, no. 1 (2011): 80–88. https://doi.org/10.1177/1099800410378889.

† Kathryn A. Lee, Mary Ellen Zaffke, and Geoffry McEnany, "Parity and Sleep Patterns during and after Pregnancy," *Obstetrics and Gynecology* 95, no. 1 (2000): 14–18, https://doi.org/10.1016/S0029-7844(99)00486-X.

gling a toddler on the playground, to keep your circadian system on track.

- If you are lactating, your sleep is more fragmented at night, but you are getting dramatically more deep sleep than usual.*
- Counterintuitively, breastfeeding at night might mean you're getting more sleep overall in the early months postpartum. Parents may get as much as forty to forty-five minutes more sleep per night if exclusively breastfeeding at night, likely because preparing bottles is more time-consuming, and because babies are less easily soothed back to sleep by the non-nursing parent.†

In practice, this is what you can do to minimize the bad news and maximize the good news:

- **Well before the baby arrives, establish your own consistent sleep-wake rhythm, eat meals at regular times, and get as much daytime light exposure as possible.** This strengthens your circadian rhythms and helps your fetus to begin learning day versus night patterns even before they're born. Don't get too rigid with all this—still listen to your body and take naps, eat snacks, and rest as needed.
- **Before the baby arrives, enlist help from as many people as possible (including daytime help).** If you have a partner living with you, come up with a tentative postpartum plan for who's go-

---

* Diane M. Blyton, C. E. Sullivan, and N. Edwards, "Lactation Is Associated with an Increase in Slow-Wave Sleep in Women," *Journal of Sleep Research* 11, no. 4 (2002): 297–303.

† Therese Doan, Annelise Gardiner, Caryl L. Gay, and Kathryn A. Lee, "Breast-Feeding Increases Sleep Duration of New Parents," *The Journal of Perinatal & Neonatal Nursing* 21, no. 3 (2007): 200–6. https://doi.org/10.1097/01.JPN.0000285809.36398.1B.

ing to be "on duty" during the night. While one person gets a few hours of uninterrupted sleep, the other will tend to the baby.*

- **When the baby arrives, know that the first month is all about survival.** Don't worry too much about so-called "good sleep habits" for you or the baby in the first few weeks (e.g., putting the baby down when they're drowsy but awake). You can start encouraging independent sleep habits later. Just be sure that you and the baby get as much sleep as possible, as long as you follow safe sleep practices for the baby, such as putting them down to sleep on their back on a flat firm surface (see the Pediatric Sleep Council's excellent website for guidelines and resources).

- **Meanwhile, try your best to return to your own circadian rhythm (and help the baby establish theirs):**
  - » Get as much daytime light exposure as possible, even if only in brief bursts of a few minutes at a time. Indoor lamps are not enough. You need sunlight on your face or a 10,000 lux light box at arm's length; even being outside on an overcast day is much better than being inside with lights on.
  - » Get active during the day (but pace yourself!†), even if it's only walking to the mailbox and back, when you're physi-

---

* For example, the plan in my household is: I will go to bed at 9:00 P.M. and sleep uninterrupted until 2:00 A.M. while my partner is "on duty" (he will nap whenever possible during this period), and he will sleep uninterrupted from 2:00 A.M. until 7:00 A.M. while I am "on duty." In reality, it probably won't be perfectly split up like this, but you get the gist. I recommend that the birth-giving parent gets the first half of the night to sleep without interruption because that's when most of their deep sleep will occur, and they need that solid sleep for physical recovery.

† I recently consulted on a case where a woman was running two to three miles per day at two weeks postpartum in order to tire herself out and sleep better. Don't do this! This soon after giving birth, your body needs to recover. Doing that much exercise is not going to help you sleep better because it will put your body on high alert. The only reason you would be running that much right after giving birth is if you're on the run from a predator, and if that's the case, your body will release more adrenaline and cortisol.

cally ready. Even puttering around the house is better than lying in bed all day, if your body is up for it.

» Minimize nighttime light exposure. Get a few warm-colored nightlights to help you safely navigate the room during night awakenings instead of turning on bright overhead lights each time.

» Minimize activity and stimulation at night. Save playtime with the baby for daytime. Keep nighttime awakenings boring and soothing.

• **If possible, try not to spend much time in your bedroom during the day.** Allow the baby to nap in a bassinet (or other safe sleep surface) outside your bedroom during the day, and do your own activities/resting outside your bedroom too. This helps both you and the baby keep days and nights separate.

• **If you decide to breastfeed (or pump breast milk), don't be afraid to do it at night.** It seems counterintuitive, but the sleep benefits of lactating may outweigh the interruption of getting up to nurse/pump.

• **As the baby begins to develop more regular nap times during the day, try your best to regularize your nap time too.** After the first month or so postpartum, try your best to not nap multiple times in a day or later than early afternoon. We want to begin returning you to your regular consolidated nighttime sleep.

• **Not everybody has to sleep in the same room at night.** If your partner's or baby's presence makes it hard for you to fall or stay asleep, which is very likely since you're naturally hypervigilant about the baby, take turns sleeping in a separate room if possible. Whoever is "on duty" sleeps in the same room as the baby, and the other person gets uninterrupted sleep elsewhere.

• **Make sure of safety, then roll with the rest.** Follow safe infant sleep practices, and make your own sleep space safe (e.g., remove tripping hazards, because you'll be disoriented and clumsy at 3:00 A.M.). Know that bizarre sleep experiences like sleep paralysis and hallucinations are likely temporary and due to severe sleep and circadian disruption that will ease in a few weeks. They're scary but won't hurt you; when they happen, just breathe, and do the 5–4–3–2–1 exercise to ground yourself to reality. Consult a sleep doctor if these symptoms are severe or last longer than a few weeks.

- **By three months postpartum, the baby should be sleeping a lot more at night than during the day** (i.e., longer bouts of sleep, shorter bouts of being awake in between), and you should also be getting the vast majority of your sleep at night. You're likely still getting up to feed the baby at night, but it should not be too difficult to fall back to sleep, and you should not be falling asleep haphazardly during the day. If this is not the case, consult a sleep specialist to assess your situation.

How Does Sleep Change During the Menopause Transition?

This question is surprisingly difficult to answer, despite menopause and sleep both being rather common occurrences for half the population. Most of the research on the topic is about sleep *disorders* during perimenopause, but there is hardly any knowledge about the normal sleep changes that one can expect during this time.* At the risk of making it seem like menopause is inherently a problem for sleep, here is what we know from the clinical research literature:

---

* My research assistant, Dr. Carol Climent, believes this is because of the medicalization of menopause—the way we collectively treat it as a women's disease instead of a normative biological experience—and I think this is an excellent point.

- Women in their late forties and early fifties are almost four times as likely to have sleep complaints as women in other age groups.*
- Over one-half of postmenopausal women have insomnia symptoms, largely due to hot flashes (and often alleviated with hormone therapy).
- When their sleep is objectively measured with polysomnography (PSG), we see that women in later perimenopause have more hyperarousal during sleep, likely due to hot flashes.†
- Women's risk of obstructive sleep apnea (OSA) goes up, with their number of apneas/hypopneas (interruptions in breathing during sleep) rising by 21 percent during early menopause and another 10 percent by late menopause.‡ Overall, postmenopausal women are three and a half times times more likely to have moderate or severe OSA than premenopausal women.§
- However, among those without sleep apnea, PSG studies have generally not found major sleep changes during menopause, suggesting that perception of sleep quality plays a role in why women feel so poorly about their sleep during this time.¶

* Hadine Joffe, Anda Massler, and Katherine M. Sharkey, "Evaluation and Management of Sleep Disturbance during the Menopause Transition," *Seminars in Reproductive Medicine* 28, no. 5 (2010): 404–21. https://doi.org/10.1055/S-0030-1262900.

† Fiona C. Baker, Laura Lampio, Tarja Saaresranta, and Päivi Polo-Kantola, "Sleep and Sleep Disorders in the Menopausal Transition," *Sleep Medicine Clinics* 13, no. 3 (2018): 443–56. https://doi.org/10.1016/J.JSMC.2018.04.011.

‡ Anna G. Mirer, Terry Young, Mari Palta, Ruth M. Benca, Amanda Rasmuson, and Paul E. Peppard, "Sleep-Disordered Breathing and the Menopausal Transition among Participants in the Sleep in Midlife Women Study," *Menopause* 24, no. 2 (2017): 157–62. https://doi.org/10.1097/GME.0000000000000744.

§ Terry Young, Laurel Finn, Diane Austin, and Andrea Peterson, "Menopausal Status and Sleep-Disordered Breathing in the Wisconsin Sleep Cohort Study," *American Journal of Respiratory and Critical Care Medicine* 167, no. 9 (2003): 1181–85. https://doi.org/10.1164/RCCM.200209-1055OC.

¶ Fiona C. Baker, Laura Lampio, Tarja Saaresranta, and Päivi Polo-Kantola, "Sleep and Sleep Disorders in the Menopausal Transition," *Sleep Medicine Clinics* 13, no. 3 (2018): 443–56. https://doi.org/10.1016/J.JSMC.2018.04.011.

This overall picture certainly seems pessimistic. But the risk factors are not entirely out of our control. I've worked with plenty of peri- and postmenopausal women who had become quite hopeless about their sleep and then became pleasantly surprised that they could restore a good relationship with it. In fact, at least one high-quality clinical trial has shown that cognitive behavioral therapy for insomnia (CBT-I), a core component of the Hello Sleep program, is effective for improving perimenopausal and postmenopausal insomnia.[*]

Here are some ways to keep things going strong with sleep during this time of hormonal upheaval:

- **All of the Hello Sleep program principles apply.** The Big Reset approaches in part II of this book are still going to be the quickest and surest way to have a physiological fresh start with sleep. Examining your relationship with sleep using approaches in part III of this book will still be your best shot to a sustainably healthy relationship with sleep.
- **Work with your healthcare team to manage vasomotor symptoms, which are major contributors to insomnia symptoms during menopause.**[†] Know that behavioral approaches can be an effective option, such as cognitive behavioral management of hot flashes and night sweats.[‡]

---

[*] Susan M. McCurry, Katherine A. Guthrie, Charles M. Morin, Nancy F. Woods, Carol A. Landis, Kristine E. Ensrud, Joseph C. Larson, et al., "Telephone-Based Cognitive Behavioral Therapy for Insomnia in Perimenopausal and Postmenopausal Women with Vasomotor Symptoms," *JAMA Internal Medicine* 176, no. 7 (July 2016): 913–920. https://doi.org/10.1001/jamainternmed.2016.1795.

[†] Ahazia Jehan, Alina Masters-Isarilov, Idoko Salifu, Ferdinand Zizi, Girardin Jean-Louis, Seithikurippu R. Pandi-Perumal, Ravi Gupta, Amnon Brzezinski, and Samy I. McFarlane, "Sleep Disorders in Postmenopausal Women," *Journal of Sleep Disorders & Therapy* 4, no. 5, 1–7 (2015). https://www.ncbi.nlm.nih.gov/pmc/articles/PMC4621258/.

[‡] Beverly Ayers, Melanie Smith, Jennifer Hellier, Eleanor Mann, and Myra S. Hunter, "Effectiveness of Group and Self-Help Cognitive Behavior Therapy in Reducing Problematic Menopausal Hot Flushes and Night Sweats (MENOS 2): A Randomized Controlled Trial," *Menopause* 19, no. 7 (July 2012): 749–59. https://doi.org/10.1097/GME.0B013E31823FE835.

- **Remember that sleep naturally changes with age and lifestyle.** It's not just hormones that change during menopause. We often also experience changes in lifestyle (e.g., activity levels), physical and mental health conditions, and social roles. Instead of expecting sleep to stay the same during all this upheaval, we can listen to our bodies' needs and be open to having healthy sleep that looks different from before.

- **Actively look out for signs and symptoms of sleep-disordered breathing (e.g., obstructive sleep apnea).** It's harder to detect sleep apnea in women because medical science on this topic, as with many others, was established by studying male patients. Err on the side of caution by talking to your doctor about snoring, daytime sleepiness, increasing blood pressure, weight gain, or waking with dry mouth or headache, especially if someone has seen you pause breathing or gasp during sleep.

- **Stay physically, mentally, and socially active.** For those of you becoming empty nesters, think of this as a second shot at your twenties. It's time to pick up hobbies, make friends, travel, and play again! You'll have fun and your sleep will thank you.

If you have yet to experience pregnancy, postpartum, or menopause, and this chapter makes you dread these seemingly inevitable dooms for sleep, know that none of them need to damage your overall relationship with sleep. After all, think of how many humans have experienced these life stages, and how many were filled with joy, wonder, and pride even against the backdrop of navigating a different sleep pattern. Good relationships can withstand change, and better yet, welcome them. As long as you continue to cherish your friend sleep and treat it with care, forgiveness, and respect, you will soon return to a happy coexistence.

BOTTOM LINE

- Pregnancy, postpartum, and menopause are times of profound hormonal, emotional, and lifestyle changes. Sleep is very often disrupted during these times.
- During pregnancy, people tend to experience much more fatigue and daytime sleepiness, more total sleep but more fragmented at night, and greater risk of sleep disorders like obstructive sleep apnea, restless legs syndrome, and frequent nightmares.
- To cope with pregnancy sleep, follow the Hello Sleep program, but be more lenient with sleep consolidation and plan to nap. Be open to sleep needs/patterns changing throughout pregnancy, go easy on yourself, and err on the side of asking your doctor about sleep apnea if there are any red flags (e.g., snoring).
- Postpartum sleep is certainly tough for the first one to three months, especially for first-time parents. The biggest challenges are interrupted nighttime sleep and flattened circadian rhythms. Fortunately, you may have a greater proportion of deep sleep, especially if you're lactating.
- To help yourself restore good sleep postpartum, try to return to a consistent sleep-wake schedule and make your days versus nights as different as possible, including getting lots of light exposure during the day and keeping things dim at night. Enlist help, and get creative about how your partner can buy you a stretch of uninterrupted sleep in the first half of the night. Make sure of safety, then roll with the rest.
- During menopause, risk for insomnia and obstructive sleep apnea rise dramatically. Vasomotor symptoms like hot flashes cause people to be more hyperaroused and sleep to be more fragmented.
- To survive the sleep challenges of the menopause transition, lean into all components of the Hello Sleep program, work with your healthcare providers to manage vasomotor symptoms, and remember to be open to changes in sleep. Err on the side of caution if you suspect signs of sleep apnea (e.g., snoring, rising blood pressure).

14

The Golden Years

How Will Sleep Change as You Get Older?

One of the biggest concerns my patients have is that sleep will get worse as they get older. In one sense, this is true, if we have a single arbitrary standard for what good sleep looks like. For example, we do tend to have less deep sleep as we age, and this certainly seems like bad news if we subscribe to an idea that more deep sleep is always better. But if we allow that change is normal, because our bodies have different needs at different times of our lives (e.g., retirees are not going through puberty, so don't need as much growth and sex hormone release as teenagers), there is nothing inherently wrong with sleep architecture taking on a different shape in older age. It's just like how our shoe size changes as we grow—we would be unhappy needing size-thirteen shoes as an adult when once we only needed size four as a child, if we arbitrarily picked size four as the perfect shoe size. Once again, it's the relationship to sleep that counts, and it is perfectly possible to maintain a great relationship with sleep into our golden years. To do so, it helps to understand what tends to change and why.

Do We Sleep Less in Older Age?

A recent study* pooling data from more than one million people from the Netherlands, the United Kingdom, and the United States has given us an excellent bird's-eye view of sleep characteristics across the lifespan, at least for people in Western countries. Researchers found that, on average, adults over the age of sixty-five get the same amount of sleep as middle-aged adults and even people in their thirties, which is seven hours per day. Their average sleep efficiency (the amount of time in bed when they were actually sleeping) was 88 percent, a percentage point or two lower than younger adults, but still solidly in the healthy range of 85 percent to 95 percent. All great news so far! These trends illustrate that sleep doesn't have to get worse as we enter retirement age, and that as a whole, older people are getting a good amount of good quality sleep.

If I Do Sleep Less as I Get Older, Will This Cause Cognitive Decline?

By now you know that averages don't tell the whole story. Just because, on average, older adults are sleeping about the same amount and at the same sleep efficiency as younger and middle-aged adults doesn't mean that *you* are. Indeed, many older adults need, and get, less sleep than they used to. But often, my patients in their sixties say, "I walked into the living room yesterday and had no idea why I went there" or "I've forgotten to get eggs from the store three times in a row!" They wonder if this is because they're sleeping less than when they were younger. There are a few things to know about this:

---

* Desana Kocevska, Thom S. Lysen, Aafje Dotinga, M. Elisabeth Koopman-Verhoeff, Maartje P. C. M. Lu- ijk, Niki Antypa, Nienke R. Biermasz, et al., "Sleep Characteristics across the Lifespan in 1.1 Million People from the Netherlands, United Kingdom and United States: A Systematic Review and Meta-Analysis," *Nature Human Behaviour* 5, no. 1 (2021): 113–22. https://doi.org/10.1038/S41562-020-00965-X.

- People of all ages misplace keys, forget names, and get confused. I, at the ripe age of thirty-three, did all three of these things today and will do so again tomorrow. You may very well be noticing these occurrences more than you did before because you're paying attention to the issue of memory decline more, so let's not yet jump to the conclusion that you have any actual cognitive impairment.*

- Even if you truly are not as sharp as you once were, we must try to accept with grace and humor that a mild amount of cognitive change is perfectly normal in healthy aging. It's okay to take a little longer to process—you've earned the leisurely pace after decades of hard work. It's also okay to forget some things—you've accumulated quite a bit more knowledge and experience than your grandkids have, and these things are competing for space in your memory stores. These changes don't necessarily have anything to do with sleep.

- Remember, sleep deprivation and sleeping less than before are different things. Most of the sensational headlines about sleep loss causing cognitive problems or accumulation of toxic materials in the brain are talking about sleep deprivation research—either animals or humans were *forcibly* kept awake in these studies. Sleeping less than before might be due to sleep deprivation, if something external is now forcing you awake, but if you're just naturally waking up earlier in the morning, this is not sleep deprivation.

- Even better news is that older adults are more resilient to sleep

---

* I had a sixty-something-year-old cancer patient become extremely concerned about dementia because a young man had walked up to her at the grocery store and offered to help, asking if she knew where she was. She concluded that she must have been so disoriented as to cause concern in a total stranger. Upon further reflection, she was not wearing her eyeglasses, so she was having to squint and take longer to find aisles thereby looking disoriented. We did a full set of neuropsychological testing, which found her to be perfectly sharp.

disruption (including real, externally induced sleep deprivation) than younger adults. They're less likely to experience negative cognitive consequences (e.g., slower reaction time) of getting less-than-usual sleep for a few nights,* and also less likely to boost new memory consolidation after sleep,† so the pressure is off. How much you sleep *tonight*, and even for a few nights this week, is neither going to help nor hinder you as much as it did decades ago.

- A few things that do correlate with cognitive function in old age are overall activity level,‡ exercise, social engagement, mental stimulation, depression, physical health, hearing changes, and health behaviors (e.g., smoking).§ These things happen to also affect sleep quality. Instead of putting all the pressure of maintaining cognitive health on controlling sleep, investing in lifestyle improvements may give you better results for both mental fitness and sleep satisfaction.

What If I've Had Insomnia in Older Age (or in the Past)? Will This Cause Dementia?

You may very well have seen headlines linking insomnia with dementia. For the purposes of highlighting the importance of sleep to mental health, these articles are not wrong to point out links between sleep and cognitive health, but if we dig deep into the original research

---

* Patricia Stenuit and Myriam Kerkhofs, "Age Modulates the Effects of Sleep Restriction in Women," *Sleep* 28, no. 10 (2005): 1283–88. https://doi.org/10.1093/SLEEP/28.10.1283.

† Michael K. Scullin and Donald L. Bliwise, "Sleep, Cognition, and Normal Aging: Integrating a Half-Century of Multidisciplinary Research," *Perspectives on Psychological Science* 10, no. 1 (2015): 97. https://doi.org/10.1177/1745691614556680.

‡ Ibid.

§ "Mild Cognitive Impairment-Symptoms and Causes-Mayo Clinic," Mayo Clinic, 2020, https://www.mayoclinic.org/diseases-conditions/mild-cognitive-impairment/symptoms-causes/syc-20354578.

that these headlines reference, we see that the data on this topic, as usual, tells a more nuanced story. The collective research conclusions are far from the "insomnia causes dementia" slam dunk that these articles proclaim. When we break down the claims about insomnia in these articles and trace them to their original sources, we find a few things:

- **They are often not really talking about insomnia.** Even in many excellent scientific publications, the terms "insomnia," "insufficient sleep," "sleep deprivation," "poor sleep quality," "sleep disturbance," and "getting less than X hours of sleep" often get used interchangeably so as to render the term "insomnia" meaningless. By now, you know that insomnia is a very specific condition: having persistent difficulty falling/staying asleep despite having ample opportunity, and feeling distressed or impaired by this problem. It's not the same thing as sleep deprivation and it's not associated with actually getting less sleep (review chapter 2 for a much more in-depth Q&A on what insomnia is and isn't).

- **They may also not be talking about dementia.** Yes, some of these studies did measure Alzheimer's disease as their main focus. But most studies' main outcomes ranged from subjective cognitive problems to mild cognitive impairment, which are much less severe than Alzheimer's disease and other forms of dementia.

- **The magnitude of findings is small.*** A recent meta-analysis (a large statistical analysis that pools data from many individual studies) found that insomnia is associated with a 27 percent increased

---

* Wei Xu, Chen Tan, Juan Zou, Xi Peng Cao, and Lan Tan, "Sleep Problems and Risk of All-Cause Cognitive Decline or Dementia: An Updated Systematic Review and Meta-Analysis," *Journal of Neurology, Neurosurgery & Psychiatry* 91, no. 3 (2020): 236–44. https://doi.org/10.1136/JNNP-2019-321896.

chance of cognitive decline. But this number decreases quite a bit if we include only the higher-quality studies that adjusted for covariates (i.e., studies that took factors like lifestyle, education level, depression, and other health conditions into account), studies that followed participants for longer periods, and studies that measured insomnia with a fine-toothed comb. In fact, in the studies that measured insomnia on a spectrum, instead of just "had it" versus "didn't have it," the association between insomnia and cognitive outcomes was zero.

- **The findings are mixed.*** Some studies have not found any link between insomnia and cognitive decline. Some have. The ones that have found a link also tend to state caveats. For example, the people with insomnia in one study were also long-term users of hypnotic sleep medications, which are known to have potential cognitive side effects. Another study found that those with insomnia *and* depression were more likely to have cognitive decline, whereas the link was less clear in those with insomnia *without* depression—and we do know that depression is associated with cognitive decline.

- **Even if there is a link, we can't tell if the chicken came before the egg.** It's impossible to do a true experiment to see if insomnia causes dementia, because that study would require researchers to give participants insomnia for a long period and see what happens to them, which is very difficult to do, not to mention unethical.† So we can only observe what naturally occurs and try to draw conclusions. This is tricky because, even if

---

* Kristine Yaffe, Cherie M. Falvey, and Tina Hoang, "Connections between Sleep and Cognition in Older Adults," *The Lancet Neurology* 13, no. 10 (2014): 1017–28. https://doi.org/10.1016/S1474-4422(14)70172-3.

† What about evidence from experimental animal research that shows a clear cause and effect? All those studies are about sleep deprivation, not insomnia, because you can sleep-deprive a rat, but you can't make it stare at the ceiling, anxiously counting the hours it has left before having to get up for work.

people with insomnia do have higher rates of dementia in old age, we can't tell if it's insomnia that causes cognitive decline, or if it's neurodegenerative disease (e.g., Alzheimer's disease) that caused insomnia in the first place, or perhaps if some third thing (say, exposure to some chemical) caused both.

- **If we work backward and look at the sleep problems in people with dementia, we see that insomnia is not the biggest issue.** Those with Alzheimer's disease or Parkinson's disease, for example, are much more likely to have excessive sleepiness (the opposite of insomnia), circadian rhythm dysfunction, and sleep-disordered breathing (e.g., sleep apnea). Yes, they also often have insomnia, but in my experience working with people with Parkinson's disease (which was the focus of my dissertation), their insomnia symptoms are much better explained by circadian dysfunction (napping a lot during the day, having no consistent rhythms).

Can I guarantee you that having had insomnia didn't increase your risk for cognitive impairment? No. There's simply no ethical way to experimentally test this. But I can assure you that whatever you've read directly linking insomnia to dementia was making research findings seem more like a slam dunk than they were, and that other factors are likely bigger risks, such as genetic risk, sedentariness, social isolation, hearing impairment, depression, other sleep disorders, etc. Bottom line, as usual: don't fret about insomnia; beef up your other health behaviors.

Why Do We Nap More in Older Age, and How Does It Affect Sleep?

If you're still worrying about sleeping less than before, don't forget that naps count as sleep, and if you're over sixty-five, you may very well be napping more than before. We know from large-scale studies that, for example, a greater percentage of Dutch, British, and American adults sixty-five and older nap (27 percent) compared to adults in the twenty-six to sixty-five age range (13.7 percent).* In part, this is because older adults have more opportunity to nap—they're more likely to be retired and not have childcare duties. If you're in your early forties, think about how often you wish you could curl up in the middle of the day but can't because you have to work, or your kids are hollering for a snack! We're also biologically more prone to napping in older age as our circadian rhythms become less robust (more on why later), so the day versus night curve is somewhat flattened: we may sleep less at night but experience more sleepiness during the day.

This is not necessarily a bad thing. Older adults who nap more or less frequently don't seem to differ on either subjective or objective overall sleep outcomes.† There are plenty of cultures, historically and in the present day, that regularly nap throughout the lifespan, and we know that regular siesta naps are a perfectly fine feature of healthy sleep. The increase in napping for older adults only becomes a problem in two scenarios:

1. **Napping haphazardly.** Accidentally falling asleep at random times and for random durations is not a good sign. It may reflect having sleep-disordered breathing (e.g., sleep apnea) or another health problem. Or it may reflect a circadian system that has lost its rhythm. The vast majority of your sleep still should happen

---

* Desana Kocevska, Thom S. Lysen, Aafje Dotinga, M. Elisabeth Koopman-Verhoeff, Maartje P. C. M. Luijk, Niki Antypa, Nienke R. Biermasz, et al., "Sleep Characteristics across the Lifespan in 1.1 Million People from the Netherlands, United Kingdom and United States: A Systematic Review and Meta-Analysis," *Nature Human Behaviour* 5, no. 1 (2021): 113–22. https://doi.org/10.1038/S41562-020-00965-X.

† Daniel J. Buysse, Kaitlin E. Browman, Timothy H. Monk, Charles F. Reynolds, Amy L. Fasiczka, and David J. Kupfer, "Napping and 24-Hour Sleep/Wake Patterns in Healthy Elderly and Young Adults," *Journal of the American Geriatrics Society* 40, no. 8 (1992): 779–86. https://doi.org/10.1111/J.1532-5415.1992.TB01849.X.

overnight. Don't let yourself get into a pattern where you end up napping in short bouts throughout the twenty-four-hour day so that your activity level, light exposure, and sleep are hardly different between day and night. Planned, regular napping is much healthier: do it at a regular time midday, and set a timer so that you don't accidentally nap for more than an hour or so.

2. **Getting frustrated about shorter nighttime sleep.** Sometimes, we want to have our cake and eat it too. We nap more during the day but still expect to sleep the same amount at night, resulting in frustration and a vicious cycle of increasing insomnia as we spend more and more time in bed trying to increase nighttime sleep that we don't need. The same principles from the Hello Sleep program still apply: you have a sleep drive piggy bank balance that you save up by being awake and active, and you can spend that balance on sleep during the day or night. It's best to spend most of it for nighttime sleep, but it's okay to budget some for a regular nap too.

Why Do We Wake Up More Often in the Night (and Earlier in the Morning)? Is Sleep Failing Us as We Get Older?

Younger adults with insomnia are more likely to have trouble falling asleep at the beginning of the night. Older adults with insomnia are more likely to have trouble staying asleep during the night. Part of this is because sleep-initiating problems self-correct in older age: older adults' circadian rhythms make them sleepy earlier in the evening, plus retired empty nesters can go to bed and get up whenever they want (I can't wait!). But there are also real changes during sleep that make older adults wake up more often and potentially have a harder time returning to sleep. These changes include:

- A greater proportion of the night is spent in lighter stages of sleep, introducing more opportunities to wake up.
- A higher rate of sleep-disordered breathing (e.g., sleep apnea, snoring) keeps sleep lighter and more fragmented.
- Other age- and health-related changes like more frequent urination, pain, and hormonal changes can also interrupt sleep.
- Lifestyle changes like lower physical activity levels, spending more time in bed, and less daytime light exposure weaken the sleep drive and circadian rhythm's ability to consolidate sleep.
- Natural circadian phase advance (a.k.a. becoming more of a biologically hardwired early bird) makes early morning awakening more common.

Most of these changes are outside of our control, so there's not too much we can do to force nighttime sleep to be more consolidated in our older age. But it's worth keeping in mind that waking up during the night (or waking earlier in the morning than you're used to) is not an inherently bad thing. Remember, even young adults wake up a dozen times or so during the night. Most older adults, even when they do wake during the night, can return to sleep pretty quickly and without much angst.

Also, whatever the reason for more frequent awakenings and lighter sleep, it doesn't make sense to be mad at your sleep's performance. Your sleep is working hard against the mounting challenges of frequent urination, hot flashes, orthopedic discomfort, apneas. If anything, we should applaud our friend sleep for its heroic efforts in the face of everything else changing. As for lighter sleep, the proportion of different sleep stages changes according to your body's needs. Young children spend at least one-quarter of the night in deep sleep (with some studies finding that they spend as much as half the night) because their bodies need this type of sleep to literally grow their bodies and brains and to learn basic things about the world at breakneck speed. Adults don't need this much deep sleep because our bodies no longer need to perform these functions, and older adults need even less because even our baseline level of bodily activity is lower. Your sleep is not failing you in older age, it's adapting to suit your needs. (But note that the above applies to generally healthy sleep in older adults. *Very* frequent awakenings due to obstructive sleep apnea or other sleep disorders are a serious problem; see below.)

Why Is Insomnia More Common in Middle and Older Age?

Even if older adults are, on average, not sleeping that much less than younger and middle-aged adults, they are more likely to experience insomnia. Why is this? Recall that sleep efficiency is one of the best indices of insomnia. Generally, if someone consistently has sleep efficiencies lower than 85 percent, they probably have insomnia. The good news is that, on average, older adults maintain good sleep efficiency that is virtually identical to younger and middle-aged adults (high 80 percent range). But interestingly, the *range* of sleep efficiencies increases a lot as we age, meaning there is much greater diversity among older adults. In other words, the older adults with the lowest sleep efficiencies are much worse off than the younger adults with the lowest sleep efficiencies. This means that something changes in the transition from middle to older adulthood for some people that causes them to spend a lot more time tossing and turning during the night. What could it be? One clue in the large Dutch-British-American study is that spending over nine hours in bed per night was significantly associated with insomnia.

This is not surprising. Remember what sleep efficiency boils down to:

$$\frac{\text{Total sleep duration}}{\text{Total time in bed}} = \text{Sleep efficiency}$$

This means you can make sleep efficiency go down in two ways: either by sleeping less or by spending more time in bed. Many of us may indeed sleep less in older adulthood because of changing biological needs and lifestyle, but this doesn't have to mean insomnia if we adapt by spending less time in bed to match our new sleep needs. This is especially important for those who have taken up napping in older age (yes, this includes accidentally dozing off in front of the TV). If you increase your amount of time in bed, that's virtually a guarantee of a lower sleep efficiency and more insomnia symptoms.

Of course, spending too much time in bed is not the only reason for insomnia in middle and older age. We've already discussed the many other changes that give insomnia more opportunity to arise (e.g., menopause, pain, nocturia). But remember also that chronic insomnia is not just about having wakefulness at night, it's about how that wakefulness affects your mood, functioning, and relationship with sleep. It's perfectly possible to have more awakenings than before, and take longer to get back to sleep, but not get pulled down the rabbit hole of anxiety and frustration about this experience.

In short, insomnia is more common among older adults, but that doesn't mean you're inevitably doomed to have insomnia in older age. All the skills you have learned in the Hello Sleep program, as well as the friendly attitude that I hope you now have about sleep, will help you to adapt to change and continue to enjoy a rich relationship with it.

Should I Be Worried About Obstructive Sleep Apnea in Older Age?

Having advocated for a "go with the flow" philosophy regarding sleep changes, I want to clarify that we should be on high alert about one thing: the dramatic rise in risk for obstructive sleep apnea (OSA) in older age. We'll dive deeper into what exactly OSA is in chapter 16. For now, suffice it to say that it involves frequent breathing interruptions during sleep, and I believe it to be one of the most underrated health problems in existence, with huge ramifications for millions of people. It's probably more common than you think, and the percentage of people who have it rises steeply with increasing age.

For example, only about 9 percent of men in their thirties have at least mild OSA, but this increases to more than one-quarter of men in their forties and fifties. For men in their sixties, a whopping 52 percent have OSA. Many of these cases are considered mild,* but about one-quarter of men in their sixties have moderately severe OSA, and close to 10 percent have severe OSA. I cannot emphasize enough how mind-boggling this is. It means that one out of ten sixty-something-year-old men stops breathing for a frighteningly long time *at least every two minutes* while they sleep. Women are less likely to have OSA, but even so, 47 percent in their sixties have at least mild OSA and 6 percent have severe OSA.

We don't fully understand why there is higher proneness to OSA in older age. Some of it may be due to weight gain, lower muscle tone, and the increasing presence of other health conditions. In any case, even if you don't think this applies to you, read the OSA section in chapter 16 and err on the side of asking your doctor about it.

What Is the Most Overlooked Sleep Change in Older Age, and Why Does This Matter Most of All?

The close reader will have already noticed that, in this chapter, I've repeatedly brought up circadian rhythms. This is the most overlooked sleep-related change in older age, and one that likely has a bigger impact

---

* In fact, such a high percentage of older adults have mild OSA that some sleep specialists consider this part of normal aging and believe we should move the threshold for OSA diagnosis higher for those over age sixty.

(other than OSA) than any of the others we've covered. Here's what usually happens to our circadian rhythms as we get older:*

- **Our circadian phase begins to shift earlier around age sixty to sixty-five**, meaning we become more biologically prone to feeling sleepy earlier in the evening and naturally waking up earlier in the morning. The circadian period also shortens with age, meaning our biological day, usually just a smidge over twenty-four hours long, shortens to less than twenty-four hours, so if left to their own devices without any way to tell time, older adults would naturally fall asleep a few minutes earlier in the evening every day. If we don't adapt to these changing biological rhythms with appropriate behavioral guardrails, along with an appropriate level of acceptance, we can spiral into insomnia.

- **We also tend to have lower circadian amplitudes.** This means that the rise and fall of rhythms—in body temperature, activity levels, hormone levels—is less dramatic throughout the twenty-four-hour cycle. The difference between the highest point and lowest point is smaller. This makes it easier for our internal clocks to be confused about the time of day / night, which means we have to work harder to give our bodies clear signals to stay on track (e.g., napping and eating meals on schedule instead of at random times).

- **The circadian system is less powerful in regulating sleep and wake.** In younger adults, the circadian system has a major say in when and how much we sleep, right alongside the equally powerful sleep drive system. That's why younger adults can

---

* Jeanne F. Duffy, Kirsi Marja Zitting, and Evan D. Chinoy, "Aging and Circadian Rhythms," *Sleep Medicine Clinics* 10, no. 4 (2015): 423–34. https://doi.org/10.1016/J.JSMC.2015.08.002.

sleep later into the morning hours, long after they've spent most of their sleep drive on the deep sleep they had in the first half of the night—their circadian drive takes over during the wee morning hours and keeps sleep going. But for older adults, their circadian system is less adept at picking up the baton for that second leg of the race, which is another reason why early-morning awakening is so common for them. On the flip side, older adults' circadian systems are also less able to keep them awake in the evenings, when their sleep drive piggy bank is getting heavy but perhaps is not yet full. That's another reason why older adults like to go to bed earlier in the evening (or even if they don't like it, they're more prone to fall asleep on the couch).

- **The brain's master clock may be getting weaker light signals from the eyes.** Recall that the brain's master clock, the suprachiasmatic nucleus (SCN; see chapter 6), can only do its job of regulating the body's rhythms well if it knows what time it is. The best clue it gets is from how much light is entering the eyes. But as eyes age, the lens is more likely to have accumulated yellow pigmentation that filters out some short wavelength light, which is specifically the type of light that stimulates the SCN. This is why we need to be extra conscientious about getting enough daytime light exposure as we age.

Do We Need to Modify Insomnia Treatment for Older Adults? Are There Any Special Tips?

The Hello Sleep program is your go-to, self-guided insomnia treatment for young, middle-, and older-aged people. I would say it's best suited for middle-aged and older adults, in part because its core components were originally designed for older adults (with the bonus that it reduces the

likelihood of depression by 50 percent for this age group).* Some of
the other components in Hello Sleep (e.g., light therapy) are especially
important as we get older. There are a couple of modifications and special considerations that can be incorporated into the program:

- For older adults with mobility problems (e.g., proneness to falling, Parkinson's disease), it may be difficult or risky to get out of
  bed unassisted during the night. If this is the case for you, modify the instruction to get out of bed when you can't fall asleep
  during the Big Reset phase. You can sit up in bed and read with
  soft lighting on, or move to a comfortable chair beside the bed
  to watch TV. The main goal is to avoid lying in bed *trying* to
  sleep, which makes your brain associate the bed with frustrating
  wakefulness and pushes sleep even farther away (conditioned
  arousal; see chapter 5).
- If you are quite sleepy during the day, give yourself a little more
  time in bed overnight and/or use a scheduled midday nap to
  help alleviate the sleepiness. If you are still sleepy even with a
  daily nap, talk to your doctor about possible OSA.
- Because of changing circadian functioning, it's extra important to get lots of light exposure during the day. Whatever activities you can do outside, do so. For example, if weather
  allows, have meals on the porch, go for a walk, read in the
  garden, etc.
- If you are experiencing worsening early morning awakening,
  modify the timing of your bright light exposure. Usually, I advocate getting a big dose of light first thing after waking up, but if

* Michael R. Irwin, Carmen Carrillo, Nina Sadeghi, Martin F. Bjurstrom, Elizabeth C. Breen, and Richard
Olmstead, "Prevention of Incident and Recurrent Major Depression in Older Adults with Insomnia: A
Randomized Clinical Trial," *JAMA Psychiatry* 79, no. 1 (November 2021): 33–41. https://doi.org/10.1001
/JAMAPSYCHIATRY.2021.3422.

you are waking up in the wee hours (e.g., 4:00 A.M.), don't blast yourself with light at least until the sun has fully risen. Too much early light exposure will push your sleep-wake timing even earlier.

- Work extra hard to avoid napping in the late afternoons and evenings. It's very easy to accidentally doze off at these times due to aging-related changes in our biology, but this will interfere with nighttime sleep. Schedule a regular siesta nap for midday instead.

- Also work extra hard on increasing your physical, social, and mental activity levels. This is not only important for your sleep, but for your mental and cognitive health. Exercise is one of the best ways to stay sharp!

- Remember that sleep and biological rhythms change with age, and it's okay. It doesn't spell doom for your relationship with sleep, nor for your cognitive health. My mantra still stands: Work *with* your biology, not against it. For example, as long as you keep your sleep-wake schedule pretty consistent, it's okay if your body naturally wants to sleep at 9:00 P.M. and wake up at 4:00 A.M. No need to force more morning hours of sleep. And it's okay to wake up several times during the night and take a few minutes to get back to sleep. Enjoy the peaceful nighttime moments and get up for some extra "me" time if these moments last longer than about thirty minutes.

- If you are experiencing cognitive impairment or depression, some of the components in Hello Sleep may feel overwhelming. Don't worry. I expound more than I need to because I want to give readers as much information as possible, but you don't actually need to do everything in this book to benefit. The biggest bang for your buck is in changing your sleep behaviors during the Big Reset (part II of this book).

BOTTOM LINE

- Sleep and circadian rhythms naturally change as we get older. The conventional wisdom is that we sleep less in older age. In reality, we might do so, but the bigger and likelier changes are shifting circadian rhythms, smaller proportion of deep sleep, and higher risk of sleep-disordered breathing (e.g., obstructive sleep apnea).

- Other than higher risk for sleep apnea, these changes are not inherently bad. We run into trouble when we expect things to stay the same and try to force arbitrary rules on our sleep patterns (e.g., resisting getting up in the morning because it seems too early).

- Having insomnia or experiencing sleep changes in older age doesn't mean you're going to get dementia. Research on this topic shows tenuous associations between insomnia and cognitive decline, whereas the facts on other factors' contribution are much stronger (e.g., exercise, physical health, social engagement).

- Something that is worth worrying about: dramatically increasing risk for obstructive sleep apnea. Please read about it in chapter 16 and err on the side of caution—talk to your doctor.

- Insomnia symptoms are more likely in older age, in large part because our sleep/circadian biology changes but our behaviors and attitudes don't adapt. The Hello Sleep program is more relevant than ever in older age.

- Very few modifications of Hello Sleep are needed for older adults. In short, you can go gentler on the Big Reset instructions if needed, but it's extra important to lean into the light + movement routine.

15

Other Medical and Psychiatric Conditions That Affect Sleep

When I saw Jorge and Maria in the sleep clinic's waiting room, I made a bet with myself that even though Jorge was the identified patient, Maria was the one who had made the appointment for him. She was sitting upright and eagerly filling out the forms, while he slouched and wore a scowl. Indeed, Jorge confessed that his wife had dragged him there. He saw little point in coming to see me ("No offense, doc") because he already knew why he had insomnia: chronic back pain. Of course he wasn't sleeping! And unless I had a magic wand to take away his pain, he couldn't fathom how seeing a sleep specialist could possibly help.

For much of this book we've approached insomnia as if it's the only health problem you have. And it might be, if you're among the minority of lucky insomniacs who don't have a comorbid medical or psychiatric condition. The truth is, most people with insomnia are like Jorge and have something else going on: pain, depression, PTSD, neurological conditions. Many medical and psychiatric conditions disrupt sleep and contribute to insomnia.

The good news is that the approaches in the Hello Sleep program work well regardless of whether you have just insomnia or other health problems as well as insomnia. In fact, the biggest research study I published was on how cognitive behavioral therapy for insomnia (CBT-I) improves not only sleep but symptoms of other disorders as well.* Comorbid conditions are often predisposing or precipitating factors for insomnia, not necessarily perpetuating factors (see chapter 2 to review the three Ps of how chronic insomnia develops; pages 51–53). Even if Jorge's sleep was initially thrown off track by his back injury, it's still mainly the conditioned arousal and disrupted sleep drive that are keeping the insomnia going now. This means we don't need a miracle cure for pain nor a time machine in order to improve his sleep.

By the end of our first appointment together, Maria was giving Jorge that "I told you so" look, and he was also more hopeful after hearing my pitch for why he was in exactly the right place. You, too, can improve your relationship with sleep through the Hello Sleep program even if you have other medical/psychiatric conditions. This chapter will briefly outline some conditions that affect sleep and what special recommendations I have for modifying insomnia therapy accordingly.

Chronic Pain, Fibromyalgia, and Arthritis

I've suffered from chronic back pain since I was a teen. Over the years particularly painful flare-ups have caused me quite a bit of anguish. I can very much empathize with those who deal with chronic pain and the ways it affects other aspects of life. When it comes to sleep, it's not a pretty picture: those with chronic pain tend to have worse sleep by every

* J. Q. Wu, E. R. Appleman, R. D. Salazar, and J. C. Ong, "Cognitive Behavioral Therapy for Insomnia Comorbid with Psychiatric and Medical Conditions a Meta-Analysis," *JAMA Internal Medicine* 175, no. 9 (2015). https://doi.org/10.1001/jamainternmed.2015.3006.

measure, and a majority have insomnia.* It's not hard to imagine why: it's difficult to find a comfortable position, the pain is distracting, and the body and brain are generally more stressed, causing hyperarousal. This is an unfortunate vicious cycle because having worse sleep can also exacerbate pain by increasing inflammation and perception of pain, as well as making it harder to emotionally cope with pain during the day.

People with fibromyalgia, a condition that involves chronic pain, along with many other symptoms, are especially likely to experience insomnia and sleep that doesn't feel restorative. This is, in part, due to very real brain activity differences during sleep. For example, people with fibromyalgia experience deep sleep that involves more alpha waves— activity that is more typical of being awake and of light sleep.† Many feel that poor sleep is the most frustrating symptom of this debilitating disorder.‡ Additionally, they don't feel that their concerns about sleep are adequately addressed by healthcare providers.§

Those with rheumatoid arthritis and osteoarthritis experience more light sleep and more insomnia symptoms as well. They may also experience more sleepiness and fatigue during the day,¶ and like those with

---

* J. L. Mathias, M. L. Cant, and A. L. J. Burke, "Sleep Disturbances and Sleep Disorders in Adults Living with Chronic Pain: A Meta-Analysis," *Sleep Medicine* 52 (December 2018): 198–210. https://doi.org/10 .1016/J.SLEEP.2018.05.023.

† Ruth M. Benca, Sonia Ancoli-Israel, Harvey, and Harvey Moldofsky, "Special Considerations in Insomnia Diagnosis and Management: Depressed, Elderly, and Chronic Pain Populations," *Journal of Clinical Psychiatry* 65, no. 8 (2004).

‡ Carolina Climent-Sanz, Genís Morera-Amenós, Filip Bellon, Roland Pastells-Peiró, Joan Blanco-Blanco, Fran Valenzuela-Pascual, and Montserrat Gea-Sánchez, "Poor Sleep Quality Experience and Self-Management Strategies in Fibromyalgia: A Qualitative Metasynthesis," *Journal of Clinical Medicine* 9, no. 12 (2020): 4000. https://doi.org/10.3390/JCM9124000.

§ Carolina Climent-Sanz, Montserrat Gea-Sánchez, Helena Fernández-Lago, José Tomás Mateos-García, Francesc Rubí-Carnacea, and Erica Briones-Vozmediano, "Sleeping Is a Nightmare: A Qualitative Study on the Experience and Management of Poor Sleep Quality in Women with Fibromyalgia," *Journal of Advanced Nursing* 77, no. 11 (2021): 4549–62. https://doi.org/10.1111/JAN.14977.

¶ Maria Eva Pickering, Roland Chapurlat, Laurence Kocher, and Laure Peter-Derex, "Sleep Disturbances and Osteoarthritis," *Pain Practice* 16, no. 2 (2016): 237–44. https://doi.org/10.1111/PAPR.12271.

other types of pain conditions, are at a much higher risk for other sleep-related disorders like obstructive sleep apnea and restless legs syndrome.

This certainly seems like a dire picture for sleep, and I won't sugarcoat things by saying that the Hello Sleep program (or any other medication or nonmedication treatment) will certainly and completely restore it to the way it was before you had chronic pain. But there is a big difference between pain and suffering. Having pain does not necessarily mean you have to suffer, and having sleep disturbance does not necessarily mean you have to struggle with insomnia. Here are some specific recommendations for getting the most out of your journey to restoring a good relationship with sleep:

- **Treat your body like a friend, not like a tool.** Thank your body for the wonderful things it allows you to do. Show compassion for your body, instead of expectation and blame. Listen to its needs and pace your activities. Feed your body the nutrition, care, and rest (not just sleep . . . but rest!) that it needs.

- **Instead of trying to escape/control the pain, sit with it.** This is the same concept as not playing tug-of-war with sleep. Once you've done what doctors have recommended to treat the condition that causes pain, what remains cannot be controlled by brute force. You may find that, by purposely bringing your non-judgmental, curious attention to the pain, you can let go of the angst and perhaps even feel less pain. See the appendix for my pain-specific mindfulness practice recommendations.

- **Spend extra time on part III of this book.** The way we think about sleep and pain plays a huge role in how we experience them. How much we struggle versus accept can have a profound effect on our bodies. See if you can apply the skills from chapters 8 and 9, especially, to your relationship with pain.

- **Take extra care to boost your circadian system.** When you have chronic pain, it's easy to spend a lot of time indoors, and to let your sleep-wake schedule fluctuate. Yes, rest is very important, and you should protect time to rest every day, but rest does not necessarily mean becoming a hermit! Get plenty of light exposure during the day, and stick to predictable rhythms, including a consistent rise time. Plan a midday nap instead of letting yourself doze whenever, wherever.

- **Be extra vigilant about possible sleep apnea and other sleep disorders.** People with chronic pain, fibromyalgia, and arthritis are much more likely to have sleep disorders (in addition to insomnia), which are likely having major impacts on your physical and mental health, including your experience of pain. Err on the side of talking to your doctor about possible signs like snoring and excessive daytime sleepiness.
- **All of the Hello Sleep program still applies.** There is no need to avoid any components, and none of them are rendered useless because you have chronic pain.

Depression and Anxiety

Mood problems are the most common co-occurring problem with insomnia: about three-quarters of those with depression also have insomnia.* In fact, many researchers believe that insomnia and mood disturbance are not just two separate things that influence each other, but rather overlapping syndromes with shared neurobiological and psychological roots.† One major hint for this overlap is that many antidepressant medications

---

* David J. Nutt, Sue Wilson, and Louise Paterson, "Sleep Disorders as Core Symptoms of Depression," *Dialogues in Clinical Neuroscience* 10, no. 3 (2008): 329–36. https://doi.org/10.31887/DCNS.2008.10.3/DNUTT.

† Ruth M. Benca and Michael J. Peterson, "Insomnia and Depression," *Sleep Medicine* 9 (2008) (SUPPL. 1): S3–9. https://doi.org/10.1016/S1389-9457(08)70010-8.

change sleep, including suppressing REM sleep,* which can counterintuitively have a mood-boosting effect. This may be why many people with
depression naturally wake up very early and can't get back to sleep. Their
brains are "self-medicating" by decreasing REM, which happens the most
during the last one-third of the night.† Another hint is that some of the
best treatment components for both depression and insomnia are the
same—bright light therapy and exercise.

When it comes to anxiety, the link may be even more obvious. For
many of my patients, one of the biggest problems with sleep is not being able to turn off worry and anxiety at night. You now know that
much of this is a conditioned arousal issue as well as an issue of not
having enough sleep drive to override the anxiety. However, it is still
true that anxiety disorders do contribute to hyperarousal.‡ On the
other hand, having sleep problems can worsen anxiety too. Disrupted
sleep, for example, can directly contribute to a more negative mood and
anxious thoughts by making the fear centers of the brain more sensitive
and reactive.§

If you're willing to have the glass-half-full perspective, this tight link
between mood and sleep is good news because it offers an opportunity
to improve two stubborn problems at the same time. In fact, we know
from meta-analysis findings that improving insomnia with cognitive

---

* Dieter Riemann and Christoph Nissen, "Sleep and Psychotropic Drugs," in *The Oxford Handbook of Sleep and Sleep Disorders*, ed. Charles Morin and Colin Espie (New York: Oxford University Press, 2012). https://doi.org/10.1093/OXFORDHB/9780195376203.013.0011.

† This does not mean you should prevent yourself from sleeping in the morning hours if you have de-pression. Your body still knows best. Depriving it of sleep that it otherwise would get is not going to help with depression.

‡ David A. Kalmbach, Andrea S. Cuamatzi-Castelan, Christine V. Tonnu, Kieulinh Michelle Tran, Jason R. Anderson, Thomas Roth, and Christopher L. Drake, "Hyperarousal and Sleep Reactivity in Insomnia: Current Insights," *Nature and Science of Sleep* 10 (2018): 193–201. https://doi.org/10.2147/NSS.S138823.

§ Andrea N. Goldstein, Stephanie M. Greer, Jared M. Saletin, Allison G. Harvey, Jack B. Nitschke, and Mat-thew P. Walker, "Tired and Apprehensive: Anxiety Amplifies the Impact of Sleep Loss on Aversive Brain Anticipation," *The Journal of Neuroscience* 33, no. 26: 10607–15. https://doi.org/10.1523/JNEUROSCI .5578-12.2013.

behavioral therapy improves depression and anxiety—two birds, one stone! Further good news: the Hello Sleep program is perfect for someone with depression/anxiety, as it includes components in addition to cognitive behavioral therapy for insomnia that are especially important for mood issues. Here are my special notes for those with depression/anxiety and insomnia:

- **Put extra effort into the light + movement portion of the Hello Sleep program (chapter 6).** Bright light exposure and physical/social activity are crucial ingredients in depression treatment. They will jumpstart the positive cycle of improving sleep and mood, allowing each to help the other.
- **Put actions ahead of thoughts.** When you're depressed/anxious, it's very hard to motivate yourself to *want* to do things, and it's very hard to have helpful, balanced thoughts. That's why you can't wait for yourself to feel like exercising, or to have optimism, before you make changes. You have to simply put one foot in front of the other and *do* it. Follow the behavioral guidelines in *Hello Sleep*, even when you don't feel like it, and allow them to jumpstart your improvement cycle.
- **Apply your pocket Socrates skills to nonsleep areas of life (chapter 8).** Track your automatic thoughts—not just the ones about sleep, but about relationships, career, health, appearance, self-worth—any area that feels stuck or hopeless. Remember that we're not trying to see things through rose-colored glasses. We're just using a system to become more aware of thoughts and to examine them with curiosity. Ask yourself if there is a more fair, accurate, and complete way to think of the situation.
- **Remember the motto, "Get out of your head and into your body" (chapters 7 and 9).** Depression and anxiety are great at digging rabbit holes for you to fall into. Use the mindfulness

skills in the Hello Sleep program day and night to get out of those and more in touch with your five senses instead. By getting in touch with reality through your body, you'll learn to shed so much unnecessary burden.

- **All of the Hello Sleep program still applies.** There is no need to avoid any of its components. None of them are rendered useless just because you have mood difficulties.

Trauma and Posttraumatic Stress Disorder

It's not surprising that experiencing trauma—events or circumstances that are extremely stressful—is detrimental to sleep. After all, sleeping is a vulnerable state, and if someone has experienced an invasive, frightening, or even life-threatening situation, the body is understandably reluctant to sink into such vulnerability. No wonder people with a trauma history are so much more likely to have insomnia and other sleep problems compared to the general population. According to the U.S. Department of Veterans Affairs, 92 percent of active duty military personnel with posttraumatic stress disorder (PTSD) and 90 percent to 100 percent of Vietnam-era veterans with PTSD have significant insomnia symptoms. Insomnia is the most common PTSD symptom for veterans of the recent wars in Afghanistan and Iraq.*

Military trauma is not the only type that causes PTSD or sleep problems. I've had patients with PTSD due to sexual trauma, motor vehicle accidents, medical events, domestic abuse, and many forms of childhood trauma. One throughline for all these patients was chronic sleep difficulty. One study, using the large adverse childhood experiences database, which includes more than seventeen thousand participants, found

---

* Philip Gehrman, *Sleep Problems in Veterans with PTSD-PTSD: National Center for PTSD*, U.S. Department of Veterans Affairs, 2020, https://www.ptsd.va.gov/professional/treat/cooccurring/sleep_problems _vets.asp.

that people who experienced more childhood stressors and traumas were much more likely to have insomnia decades later than those without these experiences.*

It breaks my heart to hear stories from my patients who have experienced trauma. Sometimes I wonder how they are able to sleep at all, given their horrendous experiences. Yet, they do sleep. It tends to feel less restful, and they have trouble falling back asleep once they wake, and some even procrastinate going to bed because they fear the inevitable nightmares . . . but sleep is such a strong basic need that their bodies do succumb almost every night, even if reluctantly. Our work together, in addition to the standard program of resetting sleep physiology and attitudes, is to teach their bodies to trust sleep again. This is difficult work, but it can be done. Multiple clinical trials have demonstrated that we can improve sleep in those who suffer from PTSD, and even better, that the PTSD itself tends to improve along the way.† One of the biggest research projects I've worked on is an ongoing clinical trial at Duke University School of Medicine where researchers are specifically treating insomnia in participants with PTSD. Here are some insights from this and other research/clinical work I've done in this area:

- **Sometimes, doing the Big Reset can be tricky for those with PTSD.** Especially for those with military or sexual trauma, going to bed can be a scary and vulnerable event. Survivors may procrastinate going to bed and end up getting very little opportunity to sleep. This means there's sometimes less flexibility

---

* Daniel P. Chapman, Anne G. Wheaton, Robert F. Anda, Janet B. Croft, Valerie J. Edwards, Yong Liu, Stephanie L. Sturgis, and Geraldine S. Perry, "Adverse Childhood Experiences and Sleep Disturbances in Adults," *Sleep Medicine* 12, no. 8 (2011): 773–79. https://doi.org/10.1016/J.SLEEP.2011.03.013.

† Fiona Yan Yee Ho, Christian S. Chan, and Kristen Nga Sze Tang, "Cognitive-Behavioral Therapy for Sleep Disturbances in Treating Posttraumatic Stress Disorder Symptoms: A Meta-Analysis of Randomized Controlled Trials," *Clinical Psychology Review* 43 (February 2016): 90–102. https://doi.org/10.1016/J.CPR.2015.09.005.

when it comes to sleep consolidation (i.e., spending less time in bed in order to increase sleep efficiency). If this is the case for you, I recommend focusing on regularizing your bed and rise times instead of curtailing your time in bed. Also, it's extra important to invest in mindfulness practice.

- **People with PTSD often don't know how to rest, even though this is especially important for them.** I see this especially often in people who had childhood trauma. Staying busy and "productive" is the only way they know how to control their environment, a crucial survival strategy during times of chaos and fear. They never learned to rest because it feels unsafe. However, they need to rest and teach their bodies that it's safe to slow down, lower their guard, and fully connect with their surroundings. This is why I would emphasize chapter 7 for readers who have experienced trauma.

- **Mindfulness can be difficult to practice, but is very important.** For many who have experienced physical/sexual abuse or life-threatening situations, being grounded in their bodies (i.e., being mindful) can feel vulnerable and unsafe. In fact, one way they might have tried to survive during trauma was to dissociate from their body. But now that you are (hopefully) not in immediate danger anymore, mindfulness is a way to teach your body to feel safe again. Start out small, with exercises like the 5–4–3–2–1 (see chapter 7, page 187) and a couple of minutes of mindful breathing per day.

- **Nightmares are treatable too.** Many people with PTSD have nightmares, sometimes about their traumatic event and sometimes about stressful things in general. No matter the content or source of these nightmares, they are more treatable than you probably realize (see chapter 16 for some brief tips, page 334). Meanwhile, don't avoid going to bed out of fear of nightmares.

Depriving yourself of sleep or disrupting the consistent timing of your sleep can actually make nightmares worse.

- **Self-compassion and patience are crucial.** Don't be mad at your body, your sleep, or your mind for giving you a hard time. They're *having* a hard time. Please be compassionate with yourself, because after everything you've been through, the last thing you need is to hear more unkind things. Treat yourself as you would an injured child. Be patient.

- **You can absolutely improve insomnia, but if PTSD is left untreated, it's hard to fully restore sleep.** This is difficult news. Plenty of research shows that we can significantly improve insomnia symptoms even when someone has had trauma. But I'll be honest, my patients with untreated PTSD often hit a wall after a decent amount of sleep improvement. There's only so far you can go with sleep when the scars of the trauma are not treated. I highly recommend working with a mental health professional trained in trauma-focused therapy—you deserve to be taken care of.

Neurodegenerative Diseases and Brain Injury

Damage to the brain profoundly impacts every aspect of our functioning, and sleep is no exception. The pathology that brings about neurodegenerative diseases like Alzheimer's and Parkinson's, for example, can start to disrupt a person's sleep years or even decades before the dementia and motor symptoms begin.* By the time Parkinson's disease is diagnosed, the vast majority of patients already have profound daytime sleepiness, insomnia, and other sleep disorders like REM behavior sleep disorder (i.e.,

---

* Aleksandar Videnovic, and Diego Golombek, "Circadian and Sleep Disorders in Parkinson's Disease," *Experimental Neurology* 243 (2013): 45–56. https://doi.org/10.1016/j.expneurol.2012.08.018.

acting out one's dreams, often violently). For people with Alzheimer's disease, too, sleep quality and quantity are significantly compromised, and more than two-thirds of them have moderate or severe obstructive sleep apnea.* One striking throughline for all different types of dementia is that circadian rhythms become much weaker: there is less difference between day and night for people's activity levels, melatonin levels, and other biological fluctuations. The neurodegeneration (i.e., breakdown of the brain) contributes to these circadian changes, and these circadian changes also exacerbate neurodegeneration.† Thankfully, researchers have found that when caregivers (family members, home care staff) are educated about the sleep health behaviors discussed in this book (e.g., light + movement, avoiding haphazard napping, etc.), people with dementia enjoy improved sleep.‡

Traumatic brain injury (TBI), too, is unkind to sleep. Both the brain injury itself and its common consequences (e.g., pain, depression, PTSD, taking many medications) can disrupt sleep, so it's unsurprising that insomnia is about five times as common for those who have experienced even mild TBI as for the general population.§ Disrupted sleep also makes it harder to heal from and cope with brain injury. Sadly, there isn't a lot of research specifically on treating insomnia for people with TBI, but the small studies that exist are quite promising: not only did cognitive behavioral therapy improve sleep, but it also improved de-

* Anna Michela Gaeta, Ivan D. Benítez, Carmen Jorge, Gerard Torres, Faride Dakterzada, Olga Minguez, Raquel Huerto, et al., "Prevalence of Obstructive Sleep Apnea in Alzheimer's Disease Patients," *Journal of Neurology* 267, no. 4 (2019): 1012–22. https://doi.org/10.1007/S00415-019-09668-4.

† Malik Nassan and Aleksandar Videnovic, "Circadian Rhythms in Neurodegenerative Disorders," *Nature Reviews Neurology* 18, no. 1 (2021): 7–24. https://doi.org/10.1038/s41582-021-00577-7.

‡ Okeanis E. Vaou, Shih Hao Lin, Chantale Branson, and Sandford Auerbach, "Sleep and Dementia," *Current Sleep Medicine Reports* 4, no. 2 (2018): 134–42. https://doi.org/10.1007/S40675-018-0112-9.

§ Jessica R. Dietch and Ansgar J. Furst, "Perspective: Cognitive Behavioral Therapy for Insomnia Is a Promising Intervention for Mild Traumatic Brain Injury," *Frontiers in Neurology* 11 (October 2020): 1208. https://doi.org/10.3389/FNEUR.2020.530273/BIBTEX.

pression symptoms and even cognitive functioning.* The challenge is, depending on how severe the brain injury and how recovery is going, mental fatigue and difficulty concentrating might make it hard to do insomnia therapy, which is sometimes mentally challenging. That's why I've included lots of checklists and fill-in-the-blank tools in this book for ease of keeping track.

My special sleep recommendations for people with neurodegenerative diseases, brain injury, and cognitive impairment are:

- **Ask your family and/or caregivers to read this book.** Chances are that if you're reading this, you *are* the caregiver, and the fact that you're taking the time to read about improving your loved one's sleep means you're doing a great job. Know that you are appreciated. Take care of your own sleep, too, using the same principles in this book, even if you don't have insomnia. Caregiving is a common precipitating factor for chronic sleep problems, so it's worth investing in some prevention now.

- **It's extra important to go outside and get light exposure during the day.** Blunted circadian rhythms are a big feature of neurodegeneration, so the brain's master clock needs extra help in keeping its rhythms strong and steady. People who have suffered brain injury are also prone to circadian problems if they are experiencing more depression and sedentariness. Resting is very important, especially if the brain injury is recent, but see if you can rest outside or by a bright window (once your doctor clears you for bright light exposure) and keep your daily rhythms consistent (e.g., sleep-wake schedule, meal schedule, appropriate level of exercise).

---

* Jessica R. Dietch and Ansgar J. Furst, "Perspective: Cognitive Behavioral Therapy for Insomnia Is a Promising Intervention for Mild Traumatic Brain Injury," *Frontiers in Neurology* 11 (October 2020): 1208. https://doi.org/10.3389/FNEUR.2020.530273/BIBTEX.

- **Take special care with fatigue and daytime sleepiness.** Most people with only insomnia and no other major medical conditions are not sleepy during the day. But with neurodegenerative disease or brain injury, daytime sleepiness and severe fatigue are common. It's absolutely okay to nap and rest! Just remember not to nap haphazardly, or to nap too long or late. Schedule a midday siesta into your daily routine. Pay extra attention to chapter 6.

- **Be patient and take baby steps.** It's okay to take your time and work gradually through the Hello Sleep program. You don't need to do a new lesson each week. Focus on one behavior change at a time: maybe start with just waking up at the same time every morning, then add staying out of the bedroom/bed during the day in order to decrease conditioned arousal, then progressively add more skills over time.

- **Use checklists and tools to keep yourself on track.** I recommend that everybody use sleep logs and the checklist tools in this book when working on insomnia, but this may be especially important for you. It's hard to remember everything!

Jorge and Maria ended up coming to insomnia therapy together and experienced excellent improvements. Much of the credit goes to Jorge. He was open-minded about treatment and did his homework. Maria's support was also crucial. In our culture, healthcare is a very individualistic domain, but sleep health can be quite dependent on other people's involvement, since a person's bed partner, daily routines, physical environment, social obligations, and many other experiences involve other people. This may be especially true for people with insomnia *and* another medical/psychiatric condition that affects sleep. **One last recommendation for everyone: share what you learned here with your loved ones, so they can know how to support you.** Sometimes a gentle reminder to go outside for a walk, or encouragement to get out of bed at your consistent rise time, can go a long way. A bonus is that they'll also stop nagging you to go to bed early if they learn that this might actually backfire and make your insomnia worse!

I'll end this chapter on an optimistic note: sleep is resilient. Yes, it is affected by trauma, depression, pain, neurodegeneration, and the many vicissitudes our bodies and minds are made to endure. But sleep is one of your staunchest supporters, and it will stick with you through the toughest of times. Your job is to support sleep back, giving it the help that it needs: consistency, gentleness, lots of daytime light, and as much investment as you can make in your physical and mental health.* Don't forget to thank your sleep for how much it does to help your healing, and to listen for what it needs from you.

---

* Remember, a good mental health professional (especially with specialized expertise in trauma, or whatever your biggest mental health need is) can change your life and is worth their weight in gold.

Other Sleep Hurdles

When Insomnia Is Not the Only Sleep Disorder You Have

You may be thinking, "Are you kidding me? Insomnia might not be the only sleep disorder I have?" Unfortunately, it's possible. There are other sleep-related disorders that can co-occur with insomnia, mimic insomnia, exacerbate insomnia, or otherwise make it harder to overcome insomnia. Knowing about them will help you understand your sleep needs, seek appropriate treatment, and modify what you do about insomnia. There is no room to cover every sleep-related disorder in detail, but I will highlight the most common and relevant ones recognized by the American Academy of Sleep Medicine's International Classification of Sleep Disorders.*

---

* American Academy of Sleep Medicine, *International Classification of Sleep Disorders*, 3rd ed. (Darien, CT: American Academy of Sleep Medicine).

Obstructive Sleep Apnea

Throughout this book, I have referred to obstructive sleep apnea (OSA) and sleep-disordered breathing, sometimes as shorthand for a whole category of sleep-related breathing disorders, which include:

- Obstructive sleep apnea (OSA) syndromes
- Central sleep apnea syndromes
- Sleep-related hypoventilation disorders
- Sleep-related hypoxemia disorder

OSA is the most common sleep-related breathing disorder. Someone with OSA experiences obstructive apneas during sleep, events during which a person stops breathing for at least ten seconds due to some physical blockage in the upper airway (e.g., relaxed tongue blocking the back of the throat). The resulting blood-oxygen drop sends alarms through the brain, forcing it to briefly wake up to breathe. An apnea usually lasts between ten and thirty seconds, but sometimes it can be over a minute long. The blood oxygen saturation level can drop by as much as 40 percent. A hypopnea is a less severe version of an apnea. Instead of a complete airway blockage, it's a partial block or one lasting fewer than ten seconds, resulting in reduced airflow. Doctors measure the severity of OSA with the apnea-hypopnea index (AHI), which represents the number of times someone has an apnea or hypopnea per hour during sleep. For example, an AHI of 5/hr means someone has, on average, five apneas/hypopneas per hour during sleep. This is considered a mild case. Severe OSA is when someone has an AHI of at least 30/hr, which means they stop breathing (or have significantly reduced airflow) at least once every two minutes. This is why people with OSA often wake up feeling unrefreshed by sleep and are sleepy during the day: their sleep was interrupted every few minutes *all night long*, and for some, this means they never reach deep sleep at all. For people who have both insomnia and OSA, the frequent awakenings caused by apneas can make the insomnia symptoms worse too. There are simply many more opportunities to wake up during the night.

OSA is not only bad for sleep quality, it also increases a person's risk of heart disease because it makes the heart work harder to oxygenate the body, which is why people with OSA are likely to have chronically high blood pressure and high heart rate, as well as increased risk for heart attacks and stroke. It can also increase risk for diabetes due to impaired glucose tolerance and insulin resistance. Because of how OSA affects sleep and brain oxygen levels, it can impair mood and cognitive performance. If OSA makes you sleepy, it also increases your risk of microsleeping at the wheel and getting into car accidents. How to know if you might be affected? Here are some risk factors and warning signs:

- Snoring, especially if loud
- Breathing pauses, gasping/snorting, or other breathing abnormalities during sleep
- Daytime sleepiness, especially if actually dozing off when not meaning to
- Waking up with dry mouth or headaches, feeling unrefreshed
- Being postmenopausal or getting into one's fifties and older
- Having unexplained high blood pressure
- Being overweight or obese
- Having a large neck size (17 inches for men, 16 inches for women)
- Smoking
- Having a family history of OSA
- Having Down syndrome
- Other conditions that cause nasal congestion or abnormal facial/head/neck bone and soft tissue structure

There are some stereotypes about OSA (e.g., it only occurs in older and obese people) that sometimes lead people to write it off as a possibility for themselves. I have worked with varsity college athletes and yoga teachers with single-digit-percentage body fat who have OSA. If you snore loudly or feel sleepy during the day even after having slept a reasonable amount, just err on the side of being safe rather than sorry.

Luckily, OSA can be treated. The standard treatment is continuous positive airway pressure (CPAP), which one of my patients has lovingly called the Darth Vader machine. It's really not that scary! CPAP involves a steady stream of air that props open the airway, delivered through a mask worn during sleep. The technology for positive airway pressure (PAP) has evolved significantly since it was invented in 1981. Nowadays, the machines are light, quiet, comfortable, and can be smart. For example, there are bi-level PAPs that ease the pressure when you exhale so it's more comfortable, and even auto-titrating PAPs that change the pressure on a breath by breath basis to deliver the least amount of air pressure needed to maintain the open airway. Other treatments include oral appliances, positional therapy (i.e., not sleeping on one's back), weight loss, and surgery. Which treatment works best depends on the severity and source of the apneas.

I know that it's a pain in the butt to get OSA diagnosed and treated. It involves seeing multiple doctors, getting an overnight sleep study, and trying out at least one new medical device that can feel intrusive in your bedroom (at least initially).* That's why 80 to 90 percent of people with OSA are not diagnosed, and an even larger percentage are untreated. This is a real shame because getting OSA treated can be a literal life-saver. I've seen again and again how a patient can go from tired, cranky, and unhealthy to feeling like they've gotten a second chance at life. My own

---

* Patients also sometimes worry that the CPAP is not sexy. But you know what else isn't sexy? Snoring like a train, having low energy, being cranky, and having higher risk for erectile dysfunction—all common consequences of OSA.

mother was diagnosed with OSA in her midfifties, and since she has started PAP treatment, she is like a new person: she's picked up hobbies, lost weight, refocused her career, traveled, found all sorts of new energy for hiking and gardening, and now she's able to watch a whole movie without falling asleep! And she's not the only one who has blossomed: our entire family is happier and healthier after the drastic improvement in our matriarch's physical and mental health. (We fight much less.)

If all of the above is still not enough incentive for you to ask your doctor about potential OSA, know that it's harder to fully treat insomnia without addressing OSA. If you hate waking up often, not being able to get back to sleep, or waking up feeling like you got run over by a truck, treating the potentially hundreds of breathing stoppages during the night is an even more important place to start than treating your insomnia.

SPECIAL CONSIDERATIONS FOR
OSA AND INSOMNIA

- **It's sometimes difficult for people to adjust to using a CPAP device.** It can feel uncomfortable, intrusive, or even cause claustrophobia or panic symptoms. Don't give up on it if you initially have a hard time. There are behavioral therapies to help you overcome barriers to using CPAP—everything from lack of motivation to severe claustrophobic responses. Look for a behavioral sleep medicine specialist to help you with these (see the appendix for provider directories).
- **It can be hard to know which to work on first—insomnia or OSA.** Sometimes it can feel like a catch-22—it's hard to improve insomnia without treating OSA, but it's also hard to use a CPAP when you already have trouble falling/staying asleep.

Personally, I would work on both at the same time. Don't wait to get OSA diagnosed and treated. At the same time, begin the Hello Sleep program (or begin insomnia treatment with a behavioral sleep medicine specialist), with special focus on keeping a consistent rise time and investing in circadian boosters (e.g., increasing bright light exposure).

- **Sometimes, OSA treatment doesn't get rid of daytime sleepiness.** In some cases, people who use their CPAP well and are benefiting from the treatment in other ways still experience daytime sleepiness. This can make insomnia treatment tricky because it's hard to stay awake in the afternoons/evenings, and haphazard or long/late naps can interfere with nighttime sleep. I recommend scheduling a regular daily nap to take the edge off without disrupting circadian rhythms or emptying your sleep drive piggy bank.

Restless Legs Syndrome and Periodic Limb Movement Disorder

Restless legs syndrome (RLS) and periodic limb movement disorder (PLMD) belong in the sleep-related movement disorders category, and both involve unusual movements of the body, usually of the limbs. When someone has RLS, they experience irresistible urges to move the legs (sometimes other body parts), usually along with unusual/uncomfortable feelings in the legs (e.g., jitters, prickles, "funny feeling"). These urges usually happen (or worsen) in the evenings/night, and are worse when sitting still or lying down, but are relieved when you move your legs.

PLMD is similar. Muscles (usually in the lower legs) twitch or tighten involuntarily, such as extension of the big toe. This mostly happens during sleep, but in severe cases it can happen during wakefulness too. The vast majority of people with RLS also have PLMD. As you can probably imagine, these involuntary movements or irresistible urges to move can make it difficult to sleep (or for your bed partner to sleep). If severe enough, they can significantly worsen sleep quality and cause daytime sleepiness/fatigue.

About 5 to 10 percent of adults have RLS, and it's about one and a half to two times more common in women. Other risk factors include:

- having iron deficiency and any medical conditions that cause iron deficiency;
- taking medications that might trigger or worsen RLS, such as Benadryl (and similar over-the-counter cold medications that contain antihistamine), antidepressants, and tranquilizers;
- being pregnant, especially if it's not a first pregnancy;
- having a family history of RLS.

Risk factors for PLMD are similar, and the biggest one is having RLS. For a lot of people with RLS and/or PLMD, treating an iron deficiency is enough to solve the problem, along with avoiding triggers and increasing the frequency of mild to moderate exercise. You will first need a ferritin test, which measures your body's iron stores and can be done as part of your regular bloodwork at a primary care clinic. It's important to note that, if you've had a ferritin test, your results might not be flagged as "too low" but you may need iron supplementation anyway. For example, the low end of "normal" for women is 11 μg/l, but if you have RLS, you may very well need treatment for levels below 75 μg/l. I would recommend showing a sleep specialist your ferritin results and discussing treatment options.

**SPECIAL CONSIDERATIONS FOR
RLS/PLMD AND INSOMNIA**

- **It is especially important to not go to bed until sleepy and to get out of bed if not sleeping.** That's because RLS symptoms are particularly bad when you're lying still, and the frustration, discomfort, and wakefulness they cause exacerbate conditioned arousal and make insomnia worse. You need to already have a *lot* of sleep drive ready to overwhelm you with sleepiness by the time you go (or go back) to bed.

- **To maximize sleep drive for bedtime, make extra effort with the light + movement component of Hello Sleep.** Getting a big dose of sunlight early in your daily routine and being active throughout the day are your best bets. You can achieve both by going for a morning walk.

- **Consider sleeping separately from your bed partner.** RLS and PLMD can disturb your bed partner's sleep, and because their sleep is fragmented, they also disturb yours. It's a vicious cycle. You both wake up unrefreshed and cranky, which is no fun.

- **Try to minimize taking Benadryl and similar over-the-counter antihistamines.** Talk to your doctor about alternatives that may be less exacerbating for your RLS.

Circadian Rhythm Sleep-Wake Disorders

In my opinion, circadian rhythm issues are underrated in the world of sleep. They cause more sleep problems than we realize but offer bigger opportunities for improving sleep too. Circadian rhythm sleep-wake disorders can be caused by brain changes, our own behaviors, or a combination of both. What they all have in common is the body's internal clocks not syncing up with environmental and social clocks (e.g., position of the sun, social obligations).

Shift Work

The International Agency for Research on Cancer has classified shift work as "probably carcinogenic."* Not to scare you, but I don't want to understate just how damaging shift work is for our health. Our brains and bodies are meant to operate on a consistent, predictable pattern: being active and awake during the day when there is broad spectrum sunlight and being inactive and/or asleep during the night when there is much less light. When we turn this pattern on its head, or worse, switch back and forth between being a daytime versus nighttime animal, we put our bodies under extreme stress. Of course, this causes sleep difficulties, which can include:

- Insomnia symptoms
- Excessive sleepiness (when one needs/wants to be awake)
- Severe fatigue
- Bizarre sleep-related symptoms (see parasomnias below)
- Sleep inertia (having difficulty getting going after waking up)

Sadly, many people—especially racial/ethnic minorities—do not have much choice when it comes to shift work. In fact, it's some of our society's most essential workers that must work unconventional shifts— healthcare workers, firefighters, law enforcement, cleaning staff, food service workers, and many more. If you are among these heroic contrib-

---

* Elizabeth M. Ward, Dori Germolec, Manolis Kogevinas, David McCormick, Roel Vermeulen, Vladimir N. Anisimov, Kristan J. Aronson et al., "Carcinogenicity of Night Shift Work," *Lancet Oncology* 20 (2019): 1058–59. https://doi.org/10.1016/S1470-2045(19)30455-3.

utors to our society, thank you. Your sacrifice makes the world go around! If you cannot, or do not want to, stop taking on shift work, here are some tips for minimizing the negative impacts on your sleep and other health:

- Try your best to not work rotating shifts. Also, make every effort to keep the same sleep-wake schedule during on- and off-work days, if possible. Get creative with your family to get enough time with them in a way that minimizes your sleep-wake schedule change throughout the week.
- If you must work rotating shifts, ask for a clockwise rotation. This means that if your shift changes, it should start later than when your previous shift started, because this pattern is easier to adjust to than starting earlier.
- Use brief naps for alertness and safety, if possible. Plan a brief nap (about thirty minutes) before or during your shift, if possible, so you are less likely to doze off when you don't mean to or make dangerous errors.
- Use sunglasses, blackout curtains, and/or eye masks to minimize light exposure leading up to and during sleep.
- Leading up to and during times when you need to function, use bright light exposure (from natural sunlight or a light box/goggles) to increase alertness.
- If you are considering switching to another job/career that would provide you with a more consistent schedule, don't forget to consider the major health benefits that come with it when you are making your decision.

Jet Lag and Social Jet Lag

Suddenly changing time zones, especially if it happens often, can simulate the effects of shift work. The change confuses your brain/body about what time it is and how it should operate. Professional basketball players have less shooting accuracy and win fewer games when they travel to play away games in a different time zone. During COVID-19, the National Basketball Association "bubbled up" all its teams in Orlando, Florida, halting travel for all. As a result, there was no home court advantage because the teams no longer had systematic circadian disruption.

Social jet lag is when you don't physically travel to a different time zone but your sleep-wake schedule changes by more than an hour or so, mimicking the effects of time zone change. For example, if you usually get up at 6:00 A.M. on weekdays but sleep in until 9:00 A.M. on weekends, you're "flying" your brain from New York to Los Angeles (and back) every week. The effects are similar to jet lag:

- Insomnia symptoms
- Daytime sleepiness
- Fatigue and sleep inertia
- Generally feeling unwell

In addition to sleep symptoms, chronic social jet lag is also associated with weight gain and obesity, depression, impaired cognitive performance, and worse metabolic and cardiovascular health.*

The best advice I have is to try to avoid frequent, unnecessary multiple-time-zone travel and to keep your sleep-wake schedule consistent seven days a week. Give yourself one hour of wiggle room (equivalent to traveling one time zone). Of course, don't avoid important or enjoyable activities like going on vacation, attending a wedding, or staying out late with friends on a Friday night just to keep your rhythms

---

* Rocco Caliandro, Astrid A. Streng, Linda W. M. Van Kerkhof, Gijsbertus T. J. Van Der Horst, and Inês Chaves, "Social Jetlag and Related Risks for Human Health: A Timely Review," *Nutrients* 13, no. 12 (2021): 4543. https://doi.org/10.3390/nu13124543.

perfect—you have to live your life too! Just balance your social needs with your circadian needs depending on what requires the most investment at this time. If you have a big trip coming up (or a major shift in your work schedule):

- During the week or so leading up to traveling, gradually adjust your sleep-wake schedule toward the schedule you'll keep in the new time zone, always leading with the easier-to-control change (e.g., going to bed later, getting up earlier) rather than the harder-to-control change (e.g., going to bed earlier with the hope of falling asleep earlier).
- Don't start adjusting too far in advance, because you don't want to live off-sync with your current time zone for much longer than you need to.
- Use sunlight or bright light to help you adjust to your new schedule. In the new time zone, spend time outside or use a light box or goggles inside during local daylight hours, especially in the local morning.

Delayed Sleep-Wake Phase Disorder and Advanced Sleep-Wake Phase Disorder

Both disorders describe a person whose biologically hardwired preference for when to sleep and wake are not "conventional" according to the majority of society. Neither are intrinsically bad, per se, but are only problematic when the mismatch between biological propensity and society's expectations clash, causing the person to function worse in their relationships or occupation.

A person with delayed sleep-wake phase is a natural night owl. The technical term is "evening chronotype." This might be you if you

- consistently have trouble falling asleep at a "decent hour";*
- would naturally sleep in later in the mornings if you didn't have obligations that forced you up at a conventional rise time;
- are a habitual snooze-button hitter, and otherwise have trouble dragging yourself out of bed on most mornings;
- feel alert, energetic, and creative in the evenings;
- have a hard time motivating yourself to go to bed at a conventional time; and
- would have great sleep quantity and quality if you were on a deserted island with no clocks and nobody expecting you to be awake during "normal" hours.

Advanced sleep-wake phase disorder (ASWPD) is similar, but you're naturally inclined to sleep and wake earlier than what most people think is normal. ASWPD is a more extreme version of having a "morning chronotype."

Delayed sleep-wake phase disorder (DSWPD) is common among teenagers and young adults. ASWPD is more common among older adults. These age-specific patterns reflect our normal, changing biology across the lifespan. Within any age group, there is natural diversity too. Some of us are hardwired to be owls, while others are hardwired to be larks, and if we go by evolutionary principles, having this diversity has probably been helpful to our species' survival.

But alas, society has arbitrary rules and stigmas that make life more difficult for those of us with unconventional chronotypes.† The consequences can be quite serious: in addition to the expected sleep prob-

---

* According to your mom, partner, society, and others who think going to bed after midnight means something is wrong with you.

† And sometimes it's not society. Sometimes it's the fact that young children are designed by some cruel god to be relentless morning people, and they come into your bedroom and literally pry open your eyelids at 6:00 A.M. "just to check if you're awake and ready to play."

lems like insomnia symptoms and daytime sleepiness/fatigue, people with DSWPD are much more likely to have depression and seasonal affective disorder, and can exacerbate symptoms of attention-deficit/hyperactivity disorder.* Here are my tips for coping as a hardwired night owl or extreme lark:

- **If possible, negotiate with your employer and loved ones to allow you a sleep-wake schedule as close to your natural inclination as possible.** For some extreme delayed sleep phase people, working second shift might be the best option. If you are privileged enough to be able to work remotely, see if you can work for a company in a different time zone that better aligns with your biology (e.g., someone with DSWPD can live in Boston and work for a company in Oregon, which allows them to get up three hours later than conventional).

- **Try your best to keep a consistent sleep-wake schedule throughout the week.** I know it's tempting to sleep in late on weekends if you're someone with a delayed chronotype, but this leads to social jet lag and makes weekdays even more difficult. Give yourself a one-hour sleeping-in allowance on weekends. If you're still sleepy, take a midday nap.

- **Use strategically timed bright light exposure.** If you're a delayed phase person, get a big dose of bright light (ideally sunlight) as soon as possible after waking, and minimize your light exposure in the evenings. If you're an advanced phase person, keep your bright lights on in the evening and don't get too much light exposure when you first wake up.

- **Talk to your doctor about using strategically timed mela-**

---

* Alexander D. Nesbitt and Derk Jan Dijk, "Out of Synch with Society: An Update on Delayed Sleep Phase Disorder," *Current Opinion in Pulmonary Medicine* 20, no. 6 (2014): 581–87. https://doi.org/10.1097/MCP .0000000000000095.

tonin in small doses. If you're a delayed phase person, taking a small daily dose of melatonin four to six hours before the desired bedtime can help to nudge your circadian phase earlier.

- **For those with DSWPD, it's especially important to have an evening wind-down ritual.** Your body needs extra help in switching gears from day to night mode, and a relaxing wind-down ritual can help to nudge along this process. If done consistently, the ritual can also help to condition an automatic response. For example, if you always dim the lights and brush your teeth leading up to bedtime, the process of doing these activities becomes associated with sleepiness, which can work like a reverse conditioned arousal.

Nightmares, Sleepwalking, and Other Parasomnias

The term "parasomnias" describes a collection of unusual sleep-related experiences that include:

- Sleepwalking, sleep talking, sleep eating, and doing other things in one's sleep
- Sleep paralysis (i.e., waking up but not being able to move)
- Sleep hallucinations (i.e., seeing/hearing things that aren't there as you're falling asleep or waking up)
- Frequent nightmares (i.e., having a very scary or upsetting dream)
- Sleep terrors, also known as night terrors (i.e., waking up with intense fear and feeling disoriented, but not from a nightmare)
- REM sleep behavior disorder (i.e., acting out dreams, often with violent behaviors like punching, kicking, running out of bed)

- Confusional arousals (i.e., waking up feeling extremely confused and acting disoriented)
- Bedwetting
- Exploding head syndrome (i.e., hearing a loud noise that doesn't exist as you're falling asleep or waking up)

Some of these symptoms have caused so much distress and superstition for people that they've given rise to all manner of paranormal beliefs. Sleep paralysis, for example, has been attributed in Japanese mythology to vengeful spirits and in Nigerian folklore to demon attacks. In modern American culture, its symptoms—the inability to move, chest pressure, feeling of doom, hallucinations—have been interpreted as experiences of alien abduction.*

These parasomnias are more common among children, becoming less common as we get older. You may experience some of these every once in a while, which is not worrisome. They can occur due to having another psychiatric/medical condition (e.g., having frequent nightmares due to PTSD, having REM sleep behavior disorder due to Parkinson's disease), sleep deprivation, severe circadian disruption, substance use, or using certain insomnia medications. Often, getting back on track with a normal sleep-wake routine, getting enough sleep, and minimizing/adjusting substances or medications will resolve the parasomnia symptoms. In rare cases, adults have persistent parasomnia symptoms even when their sleep patterns are generally good. This is a red flag for having another sleep-related disorder, such as narcolepsy, or using a medication that causes parasomnias. If any persistent parasomnia symptoms pose danger, such as sleepwalking or REM behavior sleep disorder, put safety

* José F.R. de Sá and Sérgio A. Mota-Rolim, "Sleep Paralysis in Brazilian Folklore and Other Cultures: A Brief Review," *Frontiers in Psychology* 7 (September 2016): 1–8. https://doi.org/10.3389/fpsyg.2016.01294.

measures in place to protect you and your household, such as putting up a baby gate at the top of the stairs, securing dangerous items in locked or hard-to-reach places, preventing access to fire hazards, and strongly considering sleeping separately from your bed partner.

Nightmares are the most common of parasomnias, and the most likely to be persistent in an adult without a rare sleep disorder or significantly off-track sleep habits. Frequent nightmares can happen with or without PTSD, and the recommendations are the same for both:

- Don't avoid going to bed (or otherwise curtail your opportunity to sleep) for fear of having nightmares. Keep a consistent sleep-wake schedule. Depriving yourself of sleep opportunity or having an unsteady circadian rhythm can make nightmares worse.
- When you wake from a nightmare, wake all the way up before getting back to sleep again. Use your five senses to ground yourself in reality. Get up to drink some water or use the bathroom if this helps to fully wake up.
- Practice relaxation and mindfulness exercises during the day. Give yourself plenty of time to mentally relax instead of either being in "go" mode or distracted by media consumption.
- Minimize alcohol and other psychoactive substances and review your medications with your doctor.
- Don't repeatedly replay the nightmare in your mind during the day. This may teach your brain to become more familiar with nightmare content, making it more likely to go down that path during REM sleep.
- If the above does not resolve your frequent nightmares, consult with a behavioral sleep medicine specialist about imagery rehearsal therapy, and if you have a trauma history ask

about exposure, relaxation, and rescripting therapy,* which are evidence-based treatment approaches to nightmare disorder.

Hypersomnias

Hypersomnia means being excessively sleepy. As we've seen throughout this book, hypersomnia can be caused by many things, such as not getting enough opportunity to sleep, sleep apnea and other sleep disorders, circadian disruption, certain medications, psychiatric / medical conditions, and others. This is why it's difficult to diagnose a neurological hypersomnia disorder like narcolepsy. Chances are, if you are reading a book about insomnia, you are not experiencing excessive sleepiness often, and if you are, it's most likely due to co-occurring obstructive sleep apnea or circadian disruption. But just in case insomnia is not your primary concern, or you have a loved one with unexplained excessive sleepiness, I've included a very brief primer on hypersomnias.

Narcolepsy

A debilitating neurological disorder, narcolepsy makes it very difficult to control irresistible sleepiness, which can be so overwhelming that some people experience sleep attacks, and often, even napping doesn't help for long. Some also experience sudden muscle weakness (cataplexy) that causes them to suddenly have slurred speech or even to collapse. Nighttime sleep is often compromised too, with more fragmented sleep and parasomnia symptoms like sleep paralysis and hallucinations. Many people with narcolepsy don't realize they have it, especially since it can

---

* Joanne L. Davis and David C. Wright, "Exposure, Relaxation, and Rescripting Treatment for Trauma-Related Nightmares," 7, no. 1 (2008): 5–18. https://doi.org/10.1300/J229V07N01_02.

feel like having severe insomnia plus severe daytime sleepiness, which most people don't realize is an unusual combination. To diagnose and treat narcolepsy, you would need to have a sleep study along with some daytime testing with a sleep neurologist.

Idiopathic Hypersomnia

"Idiopathic" basically means that other possible diagnoses have been ruled out and it's unclear why you have this condition. If the usual suspects that cause excessive sleepiness aren't present, it is considered idiopathic hypersomnia (IH). This disorder involves consistently sleeping much more than usual, having difficulty waking up, and still feeling unrefreshed even after a long night of sleep or a long nap, which negatively impacts functioning. Diagnosing IH involves ruling out many other possible sources of excessive sleepiness, which usually means doing a sleep study and daytime testing with a sleep neurologist. Symptoms can be managed with medication and being extra diligent about keeping a consistent sleep-wake schedule, nap scheduling, and good sleep hygiene.

One thing to note is that some people simply need more sleep than others. The range is wide between people. There are some on the extreme high end of this spectrum who function just fine if they consistently get to sleep the amount that they need. This would not be considered IH since getting enough sleep is refreshing and the longer sleep periods don't interfere with functioning.

Insufficient Sleep Syndrome

This is not so much a sleep disorder as a sleep situation—it occurs simply when someone consistently does not get enough sleep. But I cannot emphasize this enough: Insufficient sleep syndrome is *not* the same thing as insomnia. Insufficient sleep syndrome is due to a lack of opportunity to sleep. Insomnia is having enough opportunity to sleep and having trouble falling/staying asleep. See chapter 2 for an in-depth discussion about why insomnia is not synonymous with "not getting enough sleep" (pages 41–49). For people with insufficient sleep syndrome, the only way to resolve the problem is to get more opportunity to sleep.

Learning More About Sleep and Circadian Disorders

I've now covered the most common sleep and circadian rhythm disorders in each of the major diagnostic categories. As you can tell, there are many different disorders, each complex; there is much overlap between the disorders' symptoms, and they can affect each other if you have more than one. Instead of self-diagnosing, I highly recommend consulting with a healthcare provider specializing in sleep who knows the right questions to ask you in order to solve your particular sleep puzzle. When doing your own research on sleep disorders, I highly recommend sticking with one to two reputable sources (e.g., the American Academy of Sleep Medicine's website) instead of googling as much as you can and going down internet rabbit holes. There is a lot of misinformation out there, and even technically correct information can be easy to miscommunicate and misinterpret when not presented in context by professionals.

Parting Words

I hope this book has encouraged you to think about sleep as a friend, instead of a problem to be fixed. When you treat something as a friend instead of a problem, you spend more time listening with curiosity rather than imposing your will, invest in more tender care instead of rigid expectations, and are more prone to forgive than to blame. In other words, treating sleep like a friend sets you up for a healthier relationship with it in both the short and long term.

Perhaps you have already experienced the benefits of sleeping more easily. Perhaps you feel lighter, free to spend your time and energy on fulfilling things in life instead of trying to engineer your way out of insomnia. Or, perhaps, you're still working on it. That's okay—any major health change takes time, especially if you have been stuck in an unhealthy pattern for a long time or carry the burden of other health concerns too. Be patient with yourself, and give yourself credit for any progress you have made. I hope this book has given you ideas to continue pondering as well as techniques to continue practicing: one day, they may click.

These approaches represent the best clinical science we currently have about insomnia and sleep. But I must acknowledge that this science is incomplete. There is much we still need to learn, including developing insomnia therapies for people who have so far been neglected in sleep research. For example, my colleagues and I are currently wrapping up a large-scale study that scrutinizes the demographics in dozens of cognitive behavioral therapy (CBT) clinical trials for insomnia. What we're finding is that the vast majority of the participants in these trials are white, educated, affluent people living in the United States, Canada, Australia, and Western Europe. This means that, although CBT is considered the gold-standard treatment for insomnia, we don't actually know much about whether it works for the majority of the world's population.

Why wouldn't a treatment that works for one person not work for another? People who are racial/ethnic minorities in the United States, for example, often have relationships with sleep that are influenced by deep cultural wounds and intergenerational trauma. If one's ancestors were systematically sleep-deprived by those in power and literally tortured for falling asleep during the day, and if revered intellectual authorities like Thomas Jefferson himself were making a case for slavery based on slaves' tendency to nap (supposedly indicating inferior intellect),* it's hard not to feel fear and stigma toward sleep. Hence, the frequent refrain I've heard from Black patients: "I'll sleep when I'm dead." (Or, "My grandmother, the strongest person I ever knew, always said, 'I'll sleep when I'm dead.'")

There are also sweeping systemic barriers to healthy sleep for many people in the United States. As you've read in this book, the sleeping environment can directly impact sleep and circadian health: air, noise, and light pollution are not just annoyances, but real barriers to sleep for the

* Benjamin Reiss, *Wild Nights: How Taming Sleep Created Our Restless World* (New York: Basic Books, 2017).

economically disadvantaged and racially segregated who are more likely to live with them. Something like the amount of tree canopy cover in a neighborhood can predict how likely its residents are to not get enough sleep.* Shift work, which is much more common for low-wage earners and racial/ethnic minorities,† is one of the surest ways to guarantee poor sleep health. As much as we well-intentioned sleep scientists try to advocate effective treatments like CBT, light therapy, and mindfulness, it's hard enough for affluent people with flexible white-collar jobs to access these treatments and the specialists who can deliver them. People who live in rural regions or have little time/financial resources hardly stand a chance.‡

We sleep health advocates have our work cut out for us. In addition to perfecting treatments for insomnia and other sleep disorders for individual patients, we need to broaden our view. Sleep is a public health issue. Instead of placing the burden of hunting down reliable sleep information on individuals (honestly, I wouldn't know how to do that if I didn't have a PhD on this topic), we need to find big-picture ways to promote sleep health for our society:

- Designing buildings and outdoor spaces to promote more light exposure for everyone
- Arranging our work and school schedules to match children's, teens', and adults' natural circadian rhythms
- Cultivating a work culture that promotes a healthy relationship

---

* Benjamin S. Johnson, Kristen M. Malecki, Paul E. Peppard, and Kirsten M. M. Beyer, "Exposure to Neighborhood Green Space and Sleep: Evidence from the Survey of the Health of Wisconsin," *Sleep Health* 4, no. 5 (2018): 413–19. https://doi.org/10.1016/J.SLEH.2018.08.001.

† Population Reference Bureau, *A Demographic Profile of U.S. Workers Around the Clock*, September 18, 2008, https://www.prb.org/resources/a-demographic-profile-of-u-s-workers-around-the-clock/.

‡ Erin Koffel, Adam D. Bramoweth, and Christi S. Ulmer, "Increasing Access to and Utilization of Cognitive Behavioral Therapy for Insomnia (CBT-I): A Narrative Review," *Journal of General Internal Medicine* 33, no. 6 (2018): 955–62.

with rest and sleep, rather than exploiting them as resources for increasing economic output

- Protecting our environment from the calamities of climate change, which will surely impact all aspects of health, including our ability to sleep well
- Decreasing the sleep health disparities that are currently so stark

If you want to help, become an evangelist for sleep as a public health issue. Lobby your school boards about school start times, call your congressional representatives about sleep research funding, and practice role modeling appropriate boundaries at work. Tell your friends about insomnia therapy and the warning signs of obstructive sleep apnea. Let your kid nap.

Meanwhile, for your own personal sleep health, trust that sleep is a steadfast friend. And precisely because sleep is so giving and loyal, we have extra responsibility to nurture the relationship instead of taking it for granted it. This means giving your body what it needs: sunlight during the day, physical and social activity, good nutrition, moderation (and avoidance, in some cases) of psychoactive substances, and of course, proper rest. Remember to get out of your head and into your body often. Let your mind wander and explore, and not just at bedtime. Treat tiredness as a sign that your body needs something—rest, hydration, light, laughter, comfort—listen to your body without judgment, and you'll know what's needed.

With this, I wish you a strong and loving relationship with sleep—one that weathers the storms life brings, and one that brings you health and peace. Sweet dreams!

Acknowledgments

I wish to thank Dr. Ellen Hendriksen for giving me the opportunity that launched my science communication career, and the folks at Macmillan who made this book possible—especially Anna deVries, Kathy Doyle, Karen Hertzberg, Emily Miller, and Morgan Ratner.

My gratitude goes to the friends and colleagues who contributed their valuable time and expertise: Dr. Erica Appleman, Dr. Spencer Dawson, Dr. Jessica Dietch, Dr. Rachel Feuer, Dr. Justine Grosso, Dr. Abhi Jaywant, Dr. Jennifer Mundt, Dr. Gabriela Nagy, Dr. Jason Ong, Dr. Kristen Reinhardt, Dr. Clair Robbins, Dr. Alicia Roth, Dr. Paul Werth, and Dr. W. Chris Winter. Your insights have been invaluable. Thanks also to Dr. Carolina Climent Sanz and Declan McLaren for helping to make sure this book is based on the most up-to-date sleep science.

Special thanks go to the mentors whose guidance launched my career as a sleep psychologist: Dr. Alice Cronin-Golomb, Dr. Meg Danforth, Dr. Jason Ong, and Dr. Christi Ulmer. And of course, none of this would be possible without my staunchest supporter, Charlie. Thanks for holding down the fort.

Finally, my deep gratitude goes to all the patients who placed their trust in me, who helped me to grow as a clinician and scientist. I hope you continue to hold sleep as a dear friend.

Appendix

Mindfulness Resources

Learn about mindfulness:

- www.mindful.org
- Tara Brach podcast
- Books by Thich Nhat Hanh, including *The Miracle of Mindfulness*

Free guided mindfulness practice audio:

- www.mindful.org
- www.TaraBrach.com/audio
- UCLA Mindful app
- *I especially recommend mindful breathing and body scan meditations

Other apps and guides:

- Shine app (designed especially for women of color)
- Calm app
- Headspace app

Appendix

SLEEP LOG								
Complete on the morning of:		**Monday**	**Tuesday**	**Wednesday**	**Thursday**	**Friday**	**Saturday**	**Sunday**
A. Bedtime	When did you physically get into bed last night?							
B. Lights-out time	When did you start trying to sleep?							
C. Time to fall asleep (minutes)	How long did it take you to fall asleep?							
D. Number of awakenings	How many times did you wake up during the night?							
E. Time awake during the night	How long in total were you awake during the night?							
F. Wake time	When did you finally wake up for the day?							
G. Rise time	When did you physically get out of bed for the day?							
Time in bed (TiB)	(total duration from A to G)							
Total sleep time (TST)	(total duration from B to F, minus C, minus E)							
Sleep Efficiency % (SE)	TST/TiB x 100%							
Nap duration	How long did you nap yesterday?							
Any special notes?								

SLEEP LOG								
Complete on the morning of:		Monday	Tuesday	Wednesday	Thursday	Friday	Saturday	Sunday
A. Bedtime	When did you physically get into bed last night?	10:30 P.M.	10:00 P.M.	9:15 P.M.	10:45 P.M.	10:45 P.M.	11:30 P.M.	10:00 P.M.
B. Lights-out time	When did you start trying to sleep?	10:40 P.M.	10:00 P.M.	10:15 P.M.	10:45 P.M.	11:00 P.M.	11:50 P.M.	10:15 P.M.
C. Time to fall asleep (minutes)	How long did it take you to fall asleep?	30 minutes	45 minutes	60 minutes	5 minutes	10 minutes	0 minutes	10 minutes
D. Number of awakenings	How many times did you wake up during the night?	2	5	1	2	4	3	2
E. Time awake during the night	How long in total were you awake during the night?	40 minutes	75 minutes	5 minutes	10 minutes	35 minutes	60 minutes	5 minutes
F. Wake time	When did you finally wake up for the day?	5:20 A.M.	6:05 A.M.	5:45 A.M.	6:30 A.M.	5:30 A.M.	6:00 A.M.	7:15 A.M.
G. Rise time	When did you physically get out of bed for the day?	6:30 A.M.	6:30 A.M.	6:30 A.M.	6:30 A.M.	6:00 A.M.	7:30 A.M.	7:30 A.M.
Time in bed (TiB)	(total duration from A to G)	8 hours	8 hours 30 minutes	9 hours 15 minutes	7 hours 45 minutes	7 hours 15 minutes	8 hours	9 hours 30 minutes
Total sleep time (TST)	(total duration from B to F, minus C, minus E)	5 hours 30 minutes	6 hours 5 minutes	6 hours 25 minutes	7 hours 30 minutes	5 hours 45 minutes	5 hours 10 minutes	8 hours 45 minutes
Sleep Efficiency % (SE)	TST/TiB x 100%	69%	72%	69%	97%	79%	65%	92%
Nap duration	How long did you nap yesterday?	0	20 minutes	0	0	40 minutes	0	90 minutes
Any special notes?		None	Dozed while wife was driving	Stressful day	None	Accidentally fell asleep on the couch at around 10 P.M.	None	Went hiking

Appendix

Thought Record 1

Situation	Automatic Thought	Consequences (emotions, behaviors)
Can't fall asleep. It's been at least an hour.	"I won't be able to function tomorrow."	Frustrated, desperate Trying hard to relax

Thought Record 2

Situation	Automatic Thought	Consequences (emotions, behaviors)	More accurate, fair, or helpful thought	Consequences (emotions, behaviors)
Feeling tired at work	"I must have slept terribly last night."	Frustrated Annoyed	"Maybe not sleeping well is part of it, but I wonder if there's anything else making me tired."	Took a stretch, drank some water, said "hi" to a friend. Felt better.

Skills Practice Log

This can be a helpful tool for reminding yourself to practice skills learned in Hello Sleep. It's great for celebrating your efforts too!

Which skills am I working on this week?	Monday	Tuesday	Wednesday	Thursday	Friday	Saturday	Sunday
Example: Mental litter box							

Where to Find Sleep Specialists

Society of Behavioral Sleep Medicine (SBSM) Provider Directory: https://behavioralsleep.org/index.php/directory
Penn International CBT-I Provider Directory: https://cbti.directory/

Notes

- Healthcare providers are usually licensed in one state/jurisdiction, but many psychologists are now able to practice telehealth across state lines in the United States under PSYPACT (Psychology Interjurisdictional Compact), so you don't have to restrict your search to only providers in your own state. It's worth broadening your search and simply asking if someone is able to see you.
- Not all providers who practice cognitive behavioral therapy (CBT) for insomnia have the same amount of training or depth of expertise. Don't be

discouraged if the provider you chose was not a good fit. Sometimes it takes some "shopping around" to find the right one.

- For providers with the most specialized training and deepest expertise in insomnia, look for "DBSM" or "CBSM" after their names. They indicate Board of Behavioral Sleep Medicine certifications.

Self-Guided Digital Therapeutics, Websites/Apps, and Tools for Insomnia

Somryst (www.somryst.com)—A cognitive behavioral therapy for insomnia (CBT-I) digital therapeutic program requiring physician prescription. This is currently not reimbursed by health insurance.

Sleepio (www.sleepio.com)—A CBT-I digital health app. This is available through some employers.

Consensus Sleep Diary (www.consensussleepdiary.com)—A free digital sleep log app to use as a tool during and after the Hello Sleep program.

Insomnia Coach App—A free CBT-I app developed by the U.S. Veterans Administration. It includes a sleep log and educational materials about insomnia and sleep.

Where to Learn More About Sleep and Sleep Disorders

American Academy of Sleep Medicine (AASM)
https://aasm.org/clinical-resources/patient-info/

Where to Find Resources and Support for Depression, Anxiety, and PTSD

Association for Behavioral and Cognitive Therapies (ABCT)
www.abct.org/get-help

Trauma-Focused Cognitive Behavioral Therapy Directory (TF-CBT)
https://tfcbt.org/therapists

Postpartum Support International (PSI)
www.postpartum.net

Bibliography

Prologue: Sleep Is a Friend, Not an Engineering Problem

Business Communications Company, Inc. "Sleep Aids Market Size, Share & Industry Growth Analysis Report." *Market Research Reports.* January 2021. https://www.bccresearch.com/market-research/healthcare/sleep-aids-techs-markets-report.html.

Ekirch, Roger A. "Sleep We Have Lost: Pre-Industrial Slumber in the British Isles." *The American Historical Review* 106, no. 2 (2001): 343–86. https://doi.org/10.1086/AHR/106.2.343.

Ellis, Jason G., Michael L. Perlis, Laura F. Neale, Colin A. Espie, and Célyne H. Bastien. "The Natural History of Insomnia: Focus on Prevalence and Incidence of Acute Insomnia." *Journal of Psychiatric Research* 46, no. 10 (2012): 1278–85. https://doi.org/10.1016/J.JPSYCHIRES.2012.07.001.

Reiss, Benjamin. *Wild Nights: How Taming Sleep Created Our Restless World.* New York: Basic Books, 2017.

1. What Does Healthy Sleep Look Like?

Au, Jacky, and John Reece. "The Relationship between Chronotype and Depressive Symptoms: A Meta-Analysis." *Journal of Affective Disorders* 218 (August 2017): 93–104. https://doi.org/10.1016/J.JAD.2017.04.021.

Emrick, Joshua J., Brooks A. Gross, Brett T. Riley, and Gina R. Poe. "Different Simultaneous Sleep States in the Hippocampus and Neocortex." *SLEEP* 39, no. 12 (2016): 2201–9. https://doi.org/10.5665/sleep.6326.

Fan, Li, Weihao Xu, Yulun Cai, Yixin Hu, and Chenkai Wu. "Sleep Duration and the Risk of Dementia: A Systematic Review and Meta-Analysis of Prospective Cohort Studies." *Journal of the American Medical Directors Association 20, no. 12 (2019): 1480–1487. https://doi .org/10.1016/j.jamda.2019.06.009.

Gallicchio, Lisa, and Bindu Kalesan. "Sleep Duration and Mortality: A Systematic Review and Meta-Analysis." *Journal of Sleep Research* 18, no. 2 (2009): 148–58. https://doi.org/10.1111 /j.1365-2869.2008.00732.x.

Hirshkowitz, Max, Kaitlyn Whiton, Steven M. Albert, Cathy Alessi, Oliviero Bruni, Lydia DonCarlos, Nancy Hazen et al. "National Sleep Foundation's Sleep Time Duration Rec-ommendations: Methodology and Results Summary." *Sleep Health: Journal of the National Sleep Foundation* 1, no. 1 (2015): 40–43. https://doi.org/10.1016/J.SLEH.2014.12.010.

Lee-Chiong, and L. Teofilo. *Sleep: A Comprehensive Handbook*. Wilmington, DE: Wiley-Liss, 2006. https://psycnet.apa.org/record/2005-16427-000.

Nir, Yuval, Richard J. Staba, Thomas Andrillon, Vladyslav V. Vyazovskiy, Chiara Cirelli, Itzhak Fried, and Giulio Tononi. "Regional Slow Waves and Spindles in Human Sleep." *Neuron* 70, no. 1 (2011): 153–69. https://doi.org/10.1016/j.neuron.2011.02.043.

Ohara, Tomoyuki, Takanori Honda, Jun Hata, Daigo Yoshida, Naoko Mukai, Yoichiro Hi-rakawa, Mao Shibata, et al. "Association Between Daily Sleep Duration and Risk of De-mentia and Mortality in a Japanese Community." *Journal of the American Geriatrics Society* 66, no. 10 (2018): 1911–18. https://doi.org/10.1111/jgs.15446.

2. What Is Insomnia and How Did I Get It?

American Psychiatric Association. *Diagnostic and Statistical Manual-5th Edition*. 2013. https:// doi.org/10.1176/appi.books.9780890425596.744053.

Bonnet, M. H., and D. L. Arand. "Insomnia-Nocturnal Sleep Disruption-Daytime Fatigue: The Consequences of a Week of Insomnia." *Sleep* 19, no. 6 (1996): 453–461.

Harvey, Allison G., and Nicole K.Y. Tang. "(Mis)Perception of Sleep in Insomnia: A Puzzle and a Resolution." *Psychological Bulletin* 138, no. 1 (2012): 77. https://doi.org/10.1037/a0025730.

Jansen, Philip R., Kyoko Watanabe, Sven Stringer, Nathan Skene, Julien Bryois, Anke R. Hammerschlag, Christiaan A. de Leeuw et al. "Genome-Wide Analysis of Insomnia in 1,331,010 Individuals Identifies New Risk Loci and Functional Pathways." *Nature Genetics* 51, no. 3 (2019): 394–403. https://doi.org/10.1038/s41588-018-0333-3.

Miller, Christopher B., Christopher J. Gordon, Leanne Toubia, Delwyn J. Bartlett, Ronald R. Grunstein, Angela L. D'Rozario, and Nathaniel S. Marshall. "Agreement between Simple Questions about Sleep Duration and Sleep Diaries in a Large Online Survey." *Sleep Health* 1, no. 2 (2015): 133–37. https://doi.org/10.1016/J.SLEH.2015.02.007.

Spielman, A. J., L. S. Caruso, and P. B. Glovinsky. "A Behavioral Perspective on Insomnia Treat-ment." *Psychiatric Clinics of North America* 10, no. 4 (1987): 541–53. https://doi.org/10 .1016/S0193-953X(18)30532-X.

Stephan, Aurélie M., Sandro Lecci, Jacinthe Cataldi, and Francesca Siclari. "Conscious Experi-ences and High-Density EEG Patterns Predicting Subjective Sleep Depth." *Current Biology* 31, no. 24 (2021): 5487–5500.e3. https://doi.org/10.1016/J.CUB.2021.10.012.

3. Getting Ready for Your Hello Sleep Journey

Baron, Kelly Glazer, Sabra Abbott, Nancy Jao, Natalie Manalo, and Rebecca Mullen. "Orthosomnia: Are Some Patients Taking the Quantified Self Too Far?" *Journal of Clinical Sleep Medicine* 13, no. 2 (2017): 351–54. https://doi.org/10.5664/JCSM.6472.

Carney, Colleen E., Daniel J. Buysse, Sonia Ancoli-Israel, Jack D. Edinger, Andrew D. Krystal, Kenneth L. Lichstein, and Charles M Morin. "The Consensus Sleep Diary: Standardizing Prospective Sleep Self-Monitoring." *Sleep* 35, no. 2 (2012): 287–302. https://doi.org/10.5665/sleep.1642.

Edinger, Jack D., J. Todd Arnedt, Suzanne M. Bertisch, Colleen E. Carney, John J. Harrington, Kenneth L. Lichstein, Michael J. Sateia et al. "Behavioral and Psychological Treatments for Chronic Insomnia Disorder in Adults: An American Academy of Sleep Medicine Clinical Practice Guideline." *Journal of Clinical Sleep Medicine* 17, no. 2 (2021): 255–62. https://doi.org/10.5664/jcsm.8986.

Kahawage, Piyumi, Ria Jumabhoy, Kellie Hamill, Massimiliano Zambotti, and Sean P. A. Drummond. "Validity, Potential Clinical Utility, and Comparison of Consumer and Research-grade Activity Trackers in Insomnia Disorder I: In-lab Validation against Polysomnography." *Journal of Sleep Research* 29, no. 1 (2020): e12931. https://doi.org/10.1111/jsr.12931.

4. The Empty Piggy Bank: Why You Can't Fall (or Stay) Asleep

Borbély, Alexander A., Serge Daan, Anna Wirz-Justice, and Tom Deboer. "The Two-Process Model of Sleep Regulation: A Reappraisal." *Journal of Sleep Research* 25, no. 2 (2016): 131–43. https://doi.org/10.1111/JSR.12371.

Maurer, Leonie F., Colin A. Espie, Ximena Omlin, Richard Emsley, and Simon D. Kyle. "The Effect of Sleep Restriction Therapy for Insomnia on Sleep Pressure and Arousal: A Randomised Controlled Mechanistic Trial." *Sleep* 45, no 1. (January 2022): zsab223. https://doi.org/10.1093/SLEEP/ZSAB223.

Spielman, Arthur J., Paul Saskin, and Michael J. Thorpy. "Treatment of Chronic Insomnia by Restriction of Time in Bed." *Sleep* 10, no. 1 (1987): 45–56.

5. The Drooling Dog: Why Your Brain Turns "On" at Night

Bootzin, Richard R. "Stimulus Control Treatment for Insomnia." *Proceedings of the American Psychological Association* 7, no. 1 (1972): 395–396.

Harvey, Allison G., and Nicole K. Y. Tang. "(Mis)Perception of Sleep in Insomnia: A Puzzle and a Resolution." *Psychological Bulletin* 138, no. 1 (2012): 77. https://doi.org/10.1037/a0025730.

Nofzinger, Eric A., Daniel J. Buysse, Anne Germain, Julie C. Price, Jean M. Miewald, and Ba J. David Kupfer. "Functional Neuroimaging Evidence for Hyperarousal in Insomnia." *American Journal of Psychiatry* 161, no. 11 (2004): 2126–29. http://ajp.psychiatryonline.org.

Perlis, M. L., D. E. Giles, W. B. Mendelson, R. R. Bootzin, and J. K. Wyatt. "Psychophysiological Insomnia: The Behavioural Model and a Neurocognitive Perspective." *Journal of Sleep Research* 6, no. 3 (1997): 179–88. https://doi.org/10.1046/J.1365-2869.1997.00045.X.

Rehman, Ibraheem, Navid Mahabadi, Terrence Sanvictores, and Chaudhry I. Rehman. "Classical Conditioning." *Encyclopedia of Human Behavior: Second Edition* (August 2021): 484–91. https://doi.org/10.1016/B978-0-12-375000-6.00090-2.

Shechter, Ari, Elijah Wookhyun Kim, Marie Pierre St-Onge, and Andrew J. Westwood. "Blocking Nocturnal Blue Light for Insomnia: A Randomized Controlled Trial." *Journal of Psychiatric Research* 96 (January 2018): 196–202. https://doi.org/10.1016/J.JPSYCHIRES.2017.10.015.

6. Let There Be Light: The Real Answers to Fatigue (Hint: It's Not More Sleep)

Burns, Angus C., Richa Saxena, Céline Vetter, Andrew J. K. Phillips, Jacqueline M. Lane, and Sean W. Cain. "Time Spent in Outdoor Light Is Associated with Mood, Sleep, and Circadian Rhythm-Related Outcomes: A Cross-Sectional and Longitudinal Study in over 400,000 UK Biobank Participants." *Journal of Affective Disorders* 295 (January 2021): 347–52. https://doi.org/10.1016/J.JAD.2021.08.056.

de Vries, Juriena D., Madelon L. M. van Hooff, Sabine A. E. Geurts, and Michiel A. J. Kompier. "Exercise as an Intervention to Reduce Study-Related Fatigue among University Students: A Two-Arm Parallel Randomized Controlled Trial." *PloS One* 11, no. 3 (2016): 1–21. https://doi.org/10.1371/JOURNAL.PONE.0152137.

Ellingson, Laura D., Alexa E. Kuffel, Nathan J. Vack, and Dane B. Cook. "Active and Sedentary Behaviors Influence Feelings of Energy and Fatigue in Women." *Medicine and Science in Sports and Exercise* 46, no. 1 (2014): 192–200. https://doi.org/10.1249/MSS.0B013E3182A036AB.

Fortier-Brochu, Émilie, Simon Beaulieu-Bonneau, Hans Ivers, and Charles M. Morin. "Relations between Sleep, Fatigue, and Health-Related Quality of Life in Individuals with Insomnia." *Journal of Psychosomatic Research* 69, no. 5 (2010): 475–83. https://doi.org/10.1016/j.jpsychores.2010.05.005.

Golden, Robert N., Bradley N. Gaynes, R. David Ekstrom, Robert M. Hamer, Frederick M. Jacobsen, Trisha Suppes, Katherine L. Wisner, and Charles B. Nemeroff. "The Efficacy of Light Therapy in the Treatment of Mood Disorders: A Review and Meta-Analysis of the Evidence." *American Journal of Psychiatry* 162, no. 4 (2005): 656–62. https://doi.org/10.1176/APPI.AJP.162.4.656/ASSET/IMAGES/LARGE/N93F5.JPEG.

Harris, Andrea L., Nicole E. Carmona, Taryn G. Moss, and Colleen E. Carney. "Testing the Contiguity of the Sleep and Fatigue Relationship: A Daily Diary Study." *Sleep* 44, no. 5 (2021): 1–12. https://doi.org/10.1093/SLEEP/ZSAA252.

Jackson, Chandra L., Jenelle R. Walker, Marishka K. Brown, Rina Das, and Nancy L. Jones. "A Workshop Report on the Causes and Consequences of Sleep Health Disparities." *Sleep* 43, no. 8 (2020): 1–11. https://doi.org/10.1093/SLEEP/ZSAA037.

Kim, Seog Ju, Somin Kim, Sehyun Jeon, Eileen B. Leary, Fiona Barwick, and Emmanuel Mignot. "Factors Associated with Fatigue in Patients with Insomnia." *Journal of Psychiatric Research* 117 (October 2019): 24–30. https://doi.org/10.1016/j.jpsychores.2019.06.021.

Kozaki, Tomoaki, Ayaka Kubokawa, Ryunosuke Taketomi, and Keisuke Hatae. "Effects of Day-Time Exposure to Different Light Intensities on Light-Induced Melatonin Suppression at Night." *Journal of Physiological Anthropology* 34, no. 1 (2015): 1–5. https://doi.org/10.1186/S40101-015-0067-1/FIGURES/4.

Maanen, Annette van, Anne Marie Meijer, Kristiaan B. van der Heijden, and Frans J. Oort. "The Effects of Light Therapy on Sleep Problems: A Systematic Review and Meta-Analysis." *Sleep Medicine Reviews* 29 (October 2016): 52–62. https://doi.org/10.1016/J.SMRV.2015.08.009.

Ohayon, Maurice M., and Cristina Milesi. "Artificial Outdoor Nighttime Lights Associate with Altered Sleep Behavior in the American General Population." *Sleep* 39, no. 6 (2016): 1311–20. https://doi.org/10.5665/SLEEP.5860.

Schuch, Felipe B., Davy Vancampfort, Justin Richards, Simon Rosenbaum, Philip B. Ward, and Brendon Stubbs. "Exercise as a Treatment for Depression: A Meta-Analysis Adjusting for Publication Bias." *Journal of Psychiatric Research* 77 (June 2016): 42–51. https://doi.org/10.1016/J.JPSYCHIRES.2016.02.023.

Thayer, Robert E. "Energy, Tiredness, and Tension Effects of a Sugar Snack Versus Moderate Exercise." *Journal of Personality and Social Psychology* 52, no. 1 (1987): 119–25. https://doi.org/10.1037/0022-3514.52.1.119.

Wams, Emma J., Tom Woelders, Irene Marring, Laura Van Rosmalen, Domien G. M. Beersma, Marijke C. M. Gordijn, and Roelof A. Hut. "Linking Light Exposure and Subsequent Sleep: A Field Polysomnography Study in Humans." *Sleep* 40, no. 12 (2017). https://doi.org/10.1093/SLEEP/ZSX165.

7. The Mental Litter Box and Other Daytime Skills for Quieting a Racing Mind at Night

Huang, Chiung Yu, En Ting Chang, and Hui Ling Lai. "Comparing the Effects of Music and Exercise with Music for Older Adults with Insomnia." *Applied Nursing Research* 32 (November 2016): 104–10. https://doi.org/10.1016/J.APNR.2016.06.009.

Stutz, Jan, Remo Eiholzer, and Christina M. Spengler. "Effects of Evening Exercise on Sleep in Healthy Participants: A Systematic Review and Meta-Analysis." *Sports Medicine* 49, no. 2 (2019): 269–87. https://doi.org/10.1007/S40279-018-1015-0.

8. The Self-Fulfilling Prophecy: How Your Thoughts About Insomnia Feed Insomnia

Harvey, Allison G., Ann L. Sharpley, Melissa J. Ree, Katheen Stinson, and David M. Clark. "An Open Trial of Cognitive Therapy for Chronic Insomnia." *Behaviour Research and Therapy* 45, no. 10 (2007): 2491–2501. https://doi.org/10.1016/J.BRAT.2007.04.007.

9. Just Sleep, Dammit! Why Insomnia Thrives on Sleep Effort and How to Let It Go

Broomfield, Niall M., and Colin A. Espie. "Towards a Valid, Reliable Measure of Sleep Effort." *Journal of Sleep Research* 14, no. 4 (2005): 401–7. https://doi.org/10.1111/J.1365-2869.2005.00481.X.

Harris, Russ. *The Happiness Trap: How to Stop Struggling and Start Living*. Wollombi, Australia: Exisle Publishing Limited, 2008.

Hayes, Steven C. "Acceptance and Commitment Therapy, Relational Frame Theory, and the Third Wave of Behavioral and Cognitive Therapies." *Behavior Therapy* 35, no. 4 (2004): 639–65. https://doi.org/10.1016/S0005-7894(04)80013-3.

Hilton, Lara, Susanne Hempel, Brett A. Ewing, Eric Apaydin, Lea Xenakis, Sydne Newberry, Ben Colaiaco et al. "Mindfulness Meditation for Chronic Pain: Systematic Review and Meta-Analysis." *Annals of Behavioral Medicine* 51, no. 2 (2017): 199–213. https://doi.org/10.1007/S12160-016-9844-2.

Woods, H., L. M. Marchetti, S. M. Biello, and C. A. Espie. "The Clock as a Focus of Selective Attention in Those with Primary Insomnia: An Experimental Study Using a Modified Posner Paradigm." *Behaviour Research and Therapy* 47, no. 3 (2009): 231–36. https://doi.org/10.1016/J.BRAT.2008.12.009.

10. Trusting Sleep: How to Get Off Sleep Medications

Abraham, Olufunmilola, Loren J. Schleiden, Amanda L. Brothers, and Steven M. Albert. "Managing Sleep Problems Using Non-Prescription Medications and the Role of Community Pharmacists: Older Adults' Perspectives." *International Journal of Pharmacy Practice* 25, no. 6 (2017): 438–46. https://doi.org/10.1111/IJPP.12334.

Bertisch, Suzanne M., Shoshana J. Herzig, John W. Winkelman, and Catherine Buettner. "National Use of Prescription Medications for Insomnia: NHANES 1999–2010." *Sleep* 37, no. 2 (2014): 343–49. https://doi.org/10.5665/SLEEP.3410.

Brewster, Glenna, Barbara Riegel, and Philip R Gehrman. "Insomnia in the Older Adult." *Sleep Medicine Clinics* 13, no. 1 (2018): 13. https://doi.org/10.1016/J.JSMC.2017.09.002.

Edinger, Jack D., J. Todd Arnedt, Suzanne M. Bertisch, Colleen E. Carney, John J. Harrington, Kenneth L. Lichstein, Michael J. Sateia et al. "Behavioral and Psychological Treatments for Chronic Insomnia Disorder in Adults: An American Academy of Sleep Medicine Clinical Practice Guideline." *Journal of Clinical Sleep Medicine* 17, no. 2 (2021): 255–62. https://doi.org/10.5664/jcsm.8986.

Erland, Lauren A. E., and Praveen K. Saxena. "Melatonin Natural Health Products and Supplements: Presence of Serotonin and Significant Variability of Melatonin Content." *Journal of Clinical Sleep Medicine* 13, no. 2 (2017): 275. https://doi.org/10.5664/JCSM.6462.

Glass, Jennifer, Krista L. Lanctôt, Nathan Herrmann, Beth A. Sproule, and Usoa E. Busto. "Sedative Hypnotics in Older People with Insomnia: Meta-Analysis of Risks and Benefits." *BMJ : British Medical Journal* 331, no. 7526 (2005): 1169. https://doi.org/10.1136/BMJ.38623.768588.47.

Grigg-Damberger, Madeleine M., and Dessislava Ianakieva. "Poor Quality Control of Over-the-Counter Melatonin: What They Say Is Often Not What You Get." *Journal of Clinical Sleep Medicine* 13, no. 2 (2017): 163. https://doi.org/10.5664/JCSM.6434.

Hintze, Jonathan P., and Jack D. Edinger. 2020. "Hypnotic Discontinuation in Chronic Insomnia." *Sleep Medicine Clinics* 15, no. 2 (2020): 147–54. https://doi.org/10.1016/J.JSMC.2020.02.003.

Lai, L. Leanne, Mooi Heong Tan, and Yen Chi Lai. "Prevalence and Factors Associated with Off-Label Antidepressant Prescriptions for Insomnia." *Drug, Healthcare and Patient Safety* 3, no. 1 (2011): 27. https://doi.org/10.2147/DHPS.S21079.

McCall, W. Vaughn, Ralph D'Agostino, and Aaron Dunn. "A Meta-Analysis of Sleep Changes Associated with Placebo in Hypnotic Clinical Trials." *Sleep Medicine* 4, no. 1 (2003): 57–62. https://doi.org/10.1016/S1389-9457(02)00242-3.

Qaseem, Amir, Devan Kansagara, Mary Ann Forciea, Molly Cooke, and Thomas D. Denberg. "Management of Chronic Insomnia Disorder in Adults: A Clinical Practice Guideline from the American College of Physicians." *Annals of Internal Medicine* 165, no. 2 (2016): 125. https://doi.org/10.7326/M15-2175.

Sateia, Michael J., Daniel J. Buysse, Andrew D. Krystal, David N. Neubauer, and Jonathan L. Heald. "Clinical Practice Guideline for the Pharmacologic Treatment of Chronic Insomnia in Adults: An American Academy of Sleep Medicine Clinical Practice Guideline." *Journal of Clinical Sleep Medicine* 13, no. 2 (2017): 307. https://doi.org/10.5664/JCSM.6470.

Scheer, Frank A. J. L., Christopher J. Morris, Joanna I. Garcia, Carolina Smales, Erin E. Kelly, Jenny Marks, Atul Malhotra, and Steven A. Shea. "Repeated Melatonin Supplementation Improves Sleep in Hypertensive Patients Treated with Beta-Blockers: A Randomized Controlled Trial." *Sleep* 35, no. 10 (2012): 1395–1402. https://doi.org/10.5665/SLEEP.2122.

Schroder, Carmen M., Tobias Banaschewski, Joaquin Fuentes, Catherine Mary Hill, Allan Hvolby, Maj-Britt Posserud, and Oliviero Bruni. "Pediatric Prolonged-Release Melatonin for Insomnia in Children and Adolescents with Autism Spectrum Disorders." *Expert Review of Clinical Pharmacology* 22, no. 15 (2021): 2445–2454.: https://doi.org/10.1080/14656566.2021.1959549.

11. Tying Up Loose Ends: The Facts on Screens, Coffee, and Other Sleep Hygiene Topics

Babson, Kimberly A., James Sottile, and Danielle Morabito. "Cannabis, Cannabinoids, and Sleep: A Review of the Literature." *Current Psychiatry Reports* 19, no. 4 (2017): 1–12. https://doi.org/10.1007/S11920-017-0775-9.

Bolla, Karen I., Suzanne R. Lesage, Charlene E. Gamaldo, David N. Neubauer, Nae Yuh Wang, Frank R. Funderburk, Richard P. Allen, Paula M. David, and Jean Lud Cadet. "Polysomnogram Changes in Marijuana Users Who Report Sleep Disturbances during Prior Abstinence." *Sleep Medicine* 11, no. 9 (2010): 882–89. https://doi.org/10.1016/J.SLEEP.2010.02.013.

Cho, Jounhong Ryan, Eun Yeon Joo, Dae Lim Koo, and Seung Bong Hong. "Let There Be No Light: The Effect of Bedside Light on Sleep Quality and Background Electroencephalographic Rhythms." *Sleep Medicine* 14, no. 12 (2013): 1422–25. https://doi.org/10.1016/J.SLEEP.2013.09.007.

Clark, Ian, and Hans Peter Landolt. "Coffee, Caffeine, and Sleep: A Systematic Review of Epidemiological Studies and Randomized Controlled Trials." *Sleep Medicine Reviews* 31 (February 2017): 70–78. https://doi.org/10.1016/J.SMRV.2016.01.006.

Davis, J. Mark, Zuowei Zhao, Howard S. Stock, Kristen A. Mehl, James Buggy, and Gregory A. Hand. "Central Nervous System Effects of Caffeine and Adenosine on Fatigue." *American Journal of Physiology-Regulatory Integrative and Comparative Physiology* 284, no. (2003): 399–404. https://doi.org/10.1152/AJPREGU.00386.2002/ASSET/IMAGES/LARGE/H60231550004.JPEG.

Diep, Calvin, Chenchen Tian, Kathak Vachhani, Christine Won, Duminda N. Wijeysundera, Hance Clarke, Mandeep Singh, and Karim S. Ladha. "Recent Cannabis Use and Nightly Sleep Duration in Adults: A Population Analysis of the NHANES from 2005 to 2018." *Regional Anesthesia & Pain Medicine* 47 (December 2021): 100–104. https://doi.org/10.1136/RAPM-2021-103161.

Drake, Christopher, Timothy Roehrs, John Shambroom, and Thomas Roth. "Caffeine Effects on Sleep Taken 0, 3, or 6 Hours before Going to Bed." *Journal of Clinical Sleep Medicine* 9, no. 11 (2013): 1195–1200. https://doi.org/10.5664/JCSM.3170.

Drews, Henning Johannes, Sebastian Wallot, Philip Brysch, Hannah Berger-Johannsen, Sara Lena Weinhold, Panagiotis Mitkidis, Paul Christian Baier, Julia Lechinger, Andreas Roepstorff, and Robert Göder. "Bed-Sharing in Couples Is Associated With Increased and Stabilized REM Sleep and Sleep-Stage Synchronization." *Frontiers in Psychiatry* 11 (June 2020): https://doi.org/10.3389/FPSYT.2020.00583.

Dubose, Jennifer R., and Khatereh Hadi. "Improving Inpatient Environments to Support Patient Sleep." *International Journal for Quality in Health Care* 28, no. 5 (2016): 540–53. https://doi.org/10.1093/INTQHC/MZW079.

Egmond, Lieve T. van, Olga E. Titova, Eva Lindberg, Tove Fall, and Christian Benedict. "Association between Pet Ownership and Sleep in the Swedish CArdioPulmonary BioImage Study (SCAPIS)." *Scientific Reports* 11, no. 1 (2021): 1–7. https://doi.org/10.1038/S41598-021-87080-7.

Green, Amit, Merav Cohen-Zion, Abraham Haim, and Yaron Dagan. "Evening Light Exposure to Computer Screens Disrupts Human Sleep, Biological Rhythms, and Attention Abilities." *Chronobiology International* 34, no. 7 (2017): 855–865.

Irish, Leah A., Michael P. Mead, Li Cao, Allison C. Veronda, and Ross D. Crosby. "The Effect of Caffeine Abstinence on Sleep among Habitual Caffeine Users with Poor Sleep." *Journal of Sleep Research* 30, no. 1 (2021): https://doi.org/10.1111/JSR.13048.

Janků, Karolina, Michal Šmotek, Eva Fárková, and Jana Kopřivová. "Block the Light and Sleep Well: Evening Blue Light Filtration as a Part of Cognitive Behavioral Therapy for Insomnia." *Chronobiology International* 37, no. 2 (2020): 248–59. https://doi.org/10.1080/07420528.2019.1692859.

Kahn, Michal, Topi Korhonen, Leena Leinonen, Kaisu Martinmaki, Liisa Kuula, Anu Katriina Pesonen, and Michael Gradisar. "Is It Time We Stop Discouraging Evening Physical Activity? New Real-World Evidence From 150,000 Nights." *Frontiers in Public Health* 9 (November 2021): 1680. https://doi.org/10.3389/FPUBH.2021.772376/BIBTEX.

Liu, Jianghong, Tina Wu, Qisijing Liu, Shaowei Wu, and Jiu Chiuan Chen. "Air Pollution Exposure and Adverse Sleep Health across the Life Course: A Systematic Review." *Environmental Pollution* 262 (July 2020): 114263. https://doi.org/10.1016/J.ENVPOL.2020.114263.

National Center for Complementary and Integrative Health. "Cannabis (Marijuana) and Cannabinoids: What You Need To Know | NCCIH." November 2019. https://www.nccih.nih.gov/health/cannabis-marijuana-and-cannabinoids-what-you-need-to-know.

Patel, Salma I., Bernie W. Miller, Heidi E. Kosiorek, James M. Parish, Philip J. Lyng, and Lois E. Krahn. "The Effect of Dogs on Human Sleep in the Home Sleep Environment." *Mayo Clinic Proceedings* 92, no. 9 (2017): 1368–72. https://doi.org/10.1016/J.MAYOCP.2017.06.014.

Pietilë, Julia, Elina Helander, Ilkka Korhonen, Tero Myllymëki, Urho M. Kujala, and Harri Lindholm. "Acute Effect of Alcohol Intake on Cardiovascular Autonomic Regulation During the First Hours of Sleep in a Large Real-World Sample of Finnish Employees: Observational Study." *JMIR Mental Health* 5, no. 1 (2018): 1–12. https://doi.org/10.2196/MENTAL.9519.

Rångtell, Frida H., Emelie Ekstrand, Linnea Rapp, Anna Lagermalm, Lisanne Liethof, Marcela Olaya Búcaro, David Lingfors, Jan Erik Broman, Helgi B. Schiöth, and Christian Benedict. "Two Hours of Evening Reading on a Self-Luminous Tablet vs. Reading a Physical Book Does Not Alter Sleep after Daytime Bright Light Exposure." *Sleep Medicine* 23 (July 2016): 111–18. https://doi.org/10.1016/j.sleep.2016.06.016.

Salfi, Federico, Giulia Amicucci, Domenico Corigliano, Aurora D'Atri, Lorenzo Viselli, Daniela Tempesta, and Michele Ferrara. "Changes of Evening Exposure to Electronic Devices during the COVID-19 Lockdown Affect the Time Course of Sleep Disturbances." *Sleep* 44, no. 9 (2021): 1–9. https://doi.org/10.1093/SLEEP/ZSAB080.

Shahbandeh, M. "Domestic Consumption of Coffee in the United States from 2013/14 to 2019/2020." Statista. October 2020. https://www.statista.com/statistics/804271/domestic-coffee-consumption-in-the-us/.

Shechter, Ari, Elijah Wookhyun Kim, Marie Pierre St-Onge, and Andrew J. Westwood. "Blocking Nocturnal Blue Light for Insomnia: A Randomized Controlled Trial." *Journal of Psychiatric Research* 96 (January 2018): 196–202. https://doi.org/10.1016/J.JPSYCHIRES.2017.10.015.

Shechter, Ari, Kristal A. Quispe, Jennifer S. Mizhquiri Barbecho, Cody Slater, and Louise Falzon. "Interventions to Reduce Short-Wavelength ('Blue') Light Exposure at Night and Their Effects on Sleep: A Systematic Review and Meta-Analysis." *SLEEP Advances* 1, no. 1 (2020): 1–13. https://doi.org/10.1093/SLEEPADVANCES/ZPAA002.

Šmotek, Michal, Eva Fárková, Denisa Manková, and Jana Kopřivová. "Evening and Night Exposure to Screens of Media Devices and Its Association with Subjectively Perceived Sleep: Should 'Light Hygiene' Be given More Attention?" *Sleep Health* 6, no. 4 (2020): 498–505. https://doi.org/10.1016/J.SLEH.2019.11.007.

Bibliography

Steinig, Jana, Ronja Foraita, Svenja Happe, and Martin Heinze. "Perception of Sleep and Dreams in Alcohol-Dependent Patients during Detoxication and Abstinence." *Alcohol and Alcoholism* 46, no. 2 (2011): 143–47. https://doi.org/10.1093/ALCALC/AGQ087.

Thakkar, Mahesh M., Rishi Sharma, and Pradeep Sahota. "Alcohol Disrupts Sleep Homeostasis." *Alcohol* 49, no. 4 (2015): 299–310. https://doi.org/10.1016/J.ALCOHOL.2014.07.019.

12. Looking Back, Planning Ahead: How to Maintain Your Gains, Get Through Rough Patches, and Keep a Lifelong Healthy Relationship with Sleep

Ozminkowski, Ronald J., Shaohung Wang, and James K. Walsh. "The Direct and Indirect Costs of Untreated Insomnia in Adults in the United States." *Sleep* 30, no. 3 (2007): 263–73. https://doi.org/10.1093/SLEEP/30.3.263.

13. Hello Hormones! Sleep During Pregnancy, Postpartum, and Menopause

Ayers, Beverley, Melanie Smith, Jennifer Hellier, Eleanor Mann, and Myra S. Hunter. "Effectiveness of Group and Self-Help Cognitive Behavior Therapy in Reducing Problematic Menopausal Hot Flushes and Night Sweats (MENOS 2): A Randomized Controlled Trial." *Menopause* 19, no. 7 (July 2012): 749–59. https://doi.org/10.1097/GME.0B013E31823FE835.

Baker, Fiona C., Laura Lampio, Tarja Saaresranta, and Päivi Polo-Kantola. "Sleep and Sleep Disorders in the Menopausal Transition." *Sleep Medicine Clinics* 13, no. 3 (2018): 443–56. https://doi.org/10.1016/J.JSMC.2018.04.011.

Balserak, Bilgay Izci, and Kathryn Aldrich Lee. "Sleep and Sleep Disorders Associated with Pregnancy." In *Principles and Practice of Sleep Medicine*, edited by Achermann, P. and A. A. Borbély, 1525–39. New York: Elsevier, 2017.

Beck, Cheryl Tatano. "A Meta-Analysis of the Relationship between Postpartum Depression and Infant Temperament." *Nursing Research* 45, no. 4 (1996): 225–30. https://doi.org/10.1097/00006199-199607000-00006.

Christian, Lisa M., Judith E. Carroll, Douglas M. Teti, and Martica H. Hall. "Maternal Sleep in Pregnancy and Postpartum Part I: Mental, Physical, and Interpersonal Consequences." *Current Psychiatry Reports* 21, no. 3 (2019): 1–8. https://doi.org/10.1007/S11920-019-0999-Y.

Doan, Therese, Annelise Gardiner, Caryl L. Gay, and Kathryn A. Lee. "Breast-Feeding Increases Sleep Duration of New Parents." *The Journal of Perinatal & Neonatal Nursing* 21, no. 3 (2007): 200–206. https://doi.org/10.1097/01.JPN.0000285809.36398.1B.

Dunietz, Galit Levi, Wei Hao, Kerby Shedden, Claudia Holzman, Ronald D. Chervin, Lynda D. Lisabeth, Marjorie C. Treadwell, and Louise M. O'Brien. "Maternal Habitual Snoring and Blood Pressure Trajectories in Pregnancy." *Journal of Clinical Sleep Medicine* 18, no. 1 (2022): 31–38. https://doi.org/10.5664/JCSM.9474.

Gallaher, Kari Grethe Hjorthaug, Anastasiya Slyepchenko, Benicio N. Frey, Kristin Urstad, and Signe K. Dørheim. "The Role of Circadian Rhythms in Postpartum Sleep and

Mood." *Sleep Medicine Clinics* 13, no. 3 (2018): 359–74. https://doi.org/10.1016/j.jsmc
.2018.04.006.

Goyal, Deepika, Caryl Gay, and Kathryn Lee. "Fragmented Maternal Sleep Is More Strongly
Correlated with Depressive Symptoms than Infant Temperament at Three Months Post-
partum." *Archives of Women's Mental Health* 12, no. 4 (2009): 229–37. https://doi.org/10.1007
/S00737-009-0070-9/TABLES/4.

Jehan, Shazia, Alina Masters-Isarilov, Idoko Salifu, Ferdinand Zizi, Girardin Jean-Louis, Seithikurippu R. Pandi-Perumal, Ravi Gupta, Amnon Brzezinski, and Samy I. McFarlane. "Sleep Disorders in Postmenopausal Women." *Journal of Sleep Disorders & Therapy* 4, no. 5 (2015): 1–18.
https://www.ncbi.nlm.nih.gov/pmc/articles/PMC4621258/.

Joffe, Hadine, Anda Massler, and Katherine M. Sharkey. "Evaluation and Management of
Sleep Disturbance during the Menopause Transition." *Seminars in Reproductive Medicine*
28, no. 5 (2010): 404–21. https://doi.org/10.1055/S-0030-1262900.

Lee, Kathryn A., Mary Ellen Zaffke, and Geoffry McEnany. "Parity and Sleep Patterns during
and after Pregnancy." *Obstetrics & Gynecology* 95, no. 1 (2000): 14–18. https://doi.org/10
.1016/S0029-7844(99)00486-X.

McCurry, Susan M., Katherine A. Guthrie, Charles M. Morin, Nancy F. Woods, Carol A. Landis,
Kristine E. Ensrud, Joseph C. Larson et al. "Telephone-Based Cognitive Behavioral Therapy for Insomnia in Perimenopausal and Postmenopausal Women with Vasomotor Symptoms: A MsFLASH randomized clinical trial." *JAMA Internal Medicine* 176, no. 7 (2016):
913–920, https://doi.org/10.1001/jamainternmed.2016.1795.

Mirer, Anna G., Terry Young, Mari Palta, Ruth M. Benca, Amanda Rasmuson, and Paul E.
Peppard. "Sleep-Disordered Breathing and the Menopausal Transition among Participants
in the Sleep in Midlife Women Study." *Menopause* 24, no. 2 (2017): 157–62. https://doi.org
/10.1097/GME.0000000000000744.

Sedov, Ivan D., Emily E. Cameron, Sheri Madigan, and Lianne M. Tomfohr-Madsen. "Sleep
Quality during Pregnancy: A Meta-Analysis." *Sleep Medicine Reviews* 38 (April 2018): 168–176.

Stremler, R., K. M. Sharkey, and A. R. Wolfson. "Postpartum Period and Early Motherhood."
In *Principles and Practice of Sleep Medicine*, edited by Kryger, Meir H., Thomas Roth, and
William C. Dement, 1547–52. New York: Elsevier, 2017.

Suh, Sooyeon, Nayoung Cho, and Jihui Zhang. "Sex Differences in Insomnia: From Epidemiology and Etiology to Intervention." *Current Psychiatry Reports* 20, no. 9 (2018): 1–12.
https://doi.org/10.1007/S11920-018-0940-9.

Thomas, Karen A., and Robert L. Burr. "Melatonin Level and Pattern in Postpartum Versus
Nonpregnant Nulliparous Women." *Journal of Obstetric, Gynecologic & Neonatal Nursing*
35, no. 5 (2006): 608–15. https://doi.org/10.1111/J.1552-6909.2006.00082.X.

Tsai, Shao Yu, Kathryn E. Barnard, Martha J. Lentz, and Karen A. Thomas. "Mother-Infant
Activity Synchrony as a Correlate of the Emergence of Circadian Rhythm." *Biological
Research for Nursing* 13, no. 1 (2011): 80–88. https://doi.org/10.1177/1099800410378889.

Won, Christine H. J. "Sleeping for Two: The Great Paradox of Sleep in Pregnancy." *Journal of
Clinical Sleep Medicine* 11, no. 6 (2015): 593–94. https://doi.org/10.5664/JCSM.4760.

Young, Terry, Laurel Finn, Diane Austin, and Andrea Peterson. "Menopausal Status and Sleep-Disordered Breathing in the Wisconsin Sleep Cohort Study." *American Journal of Respiratory and Critical Care Medicine* 167, no. 9 (2003): 1181–85. https://doi.org/10.1164/RCCM .200209-1055OC.

Zhang, Jihui, Ngan Yin Chan, Siu Ping Lam, Shirley Xin Li, Yaping Liu, Joey W. Y. Chan, Alice Pik Shan Kong, et al. "Emergence of Sex Differences in Insomnia Symptoms in Adolescents: A Large-Scale School-Based Study." *Sleep* 39, no. 8 (2016): 1563–70. https://doi .org/10.5665/SLEEP.6022.

14. The Golden Years: How Will Sleep Change as You Get Older?

Buysse, Daniel J., Kaitlin E. Browman, Timothy H. Monk, Charles F. Reynolds, Amy L. Fasiczka, and David J. Kupfer. "Napping and 24-Hour Sleep/Wake Patterns in Healthy Elderly and Young Adults." *Journal of the American Geriatrics Society* 40, no. 8 (1992): 779–86. https://doi.org/10.1111/J.1532-5415.1992.TB01849.X.

Dause, Tyler, and Elizabeth Kirby. "Aging Gracefully: Social Engagement Joins Exercise and Enrichment as a Key Lifestyle Factor in Resistance to Age-Related Cognitive Decline." *Neural Regeneration Research* 14, no. 1 (2019): 39. https://doi.org/10.4103/1673-5374.243698.

Duffy, Jeanne F., Kirsi Marja Zitting, and Evan D. Chinoy. "Aging and Circadian Rhythms." *Sleep Medicine Clinics* 10, no. 4 (2015): 423–34. https://doi.org/10.1016/J.JSMC.2015.08 .002.

Durán, Joaquin, Santiago Esnaola, Ramón Rubio, and Ángeles Iztueta. "Obstructive Sleep Apnea-Hypopnea and Related Clinical Features in a Population-Based Sample of Subjects Aged 30 to 70 Yr." *American Journal of Respiratory and Critical Care Medicine* 163, (3 Pt 1) (2001): 685–89. https://doi.org/10.1164/AJRCCM.163.3.2005065.

Irwin, Michael R., Carmen Carrillo, Nina Sadeghi, Martin F. Bjurstrom, Elizabeth C. Breen, and Richard Olmstead. "Prevention of Incident and Recurrent Major Depression in Older Adults with Insomnia: A Randomized Clinical Trial." *JAMA Psychiatry* 79, no. 1 (2022): 33–41, https://doi.org/10.1001/JAMAPSYCHIATRY.2021.3422.

Kocevska, Desana, Thom S. Lysen, Aafje Dotinga, M. Elisabeth Koopman-Verhoeff, Maartje P. C. M. Luijk, Niki Antypa, Nienke R. Biermasz, et al. "Sleep Characteristics across the Lifespan in 1.1 Million People from the Netherlands, United Kingdom and United States: A Systematic Review and Meta-Analysis." *Nature Human Behaviour* 5, no. 1 (2021): 113–22. https://doi.org/10.1038/S41562-020-00965-X.

"Mild Cognitive Impairment-Symptoms and Causes-Mayo Clinic." Mayo Clinic. https://www .mayoclinic.org/diseases-conditions/mild-cognitive-impairment/symptoms-causes/syc -20354578.

Ohayon, Maurice M., Mary A. Carskadon, Christian Guilleminault, and Michael V. Vitiello. "Meta-Analysis of Quantitative Sleep Parameters From Childhood to Old Age in Healthy Individuals: Developing Normative Sleep Values Across the Human Lifespan." *Sleep* 27, no. 7 (2004): 1255–73. https://doi.org/10.1093/SLEEP/27.7.1255.

Scullin, Michael K., and Donald L. Bliwise. "Sleep, Cognition, and Normal Aging: Integrating a Half-Century of Multidisciplinary Research." *Perspectives on Psychological Science: A Journal of the Association for Psychological Science* 10, no. 1 (2015): 97. https://doi.org/10.1177 /1745691614556680.

Stenuit, Patricia, and Myriam Kerkhofs. "Age Modulates the Effects of Sleep Restriction in Women." *Sleep* 28, no. 10 (2005): 1283–88. https://doi.org/10.1093/SLEEP/28.10 .1283.

Xu, Wei, Chen Chen Tan, Juan Juan Zou, Xi Peng Cao, and Lan Tan. "Sleep Problems and Risk of All-Cause Cognitive Decline or Dementia: An Updated Systematic Review and Meta-Analysis." *Journal of Neurology, Neurosurgery & Psychiatry* 91, no. 3 (2020): 236–44. https://doi.org/10.1136/JNNP-2019-321896.

Yaffe, Kristine, Cherie M. Falvey, and Tina Hoang. "Connections between Sleep and Cognition in Older Adults." *The Lancet Neurology* 13, no. 10 (2014): 1017–28. https://doi.org/10.1016 /S1474-4422(14)70172-3.

15. Other Medical and Psychiatric Conditions That Affect Sleep

Benca, Ruth M., and Michael J. Peterson. "Insomnia and Depression." *Sleep Medicine* 9, no. 1 (2008): S3–9. https://doi.org/10.1016/S1389-9457(08)70010-8.

Benca, Ruth M., Sonia Ancoli-Israel, and Harvey Moldofsky. "Special Considerations in Insomnia Diagnosis and Management: Depressed, Elderly, and Chronic Pain Populations." *Journal of Clinical Psychiatry* 65, no. 8 (2004) 26–35.

Chapman, Daniel P., Anne G. Wheaton, Robert F. Anda, Janet B. Croft, Valerie J. Edwards, Yong Liu, Stephanie L. Sturgis, and Geraldine S. Perry. "Adverse Childhood Experiences and Sleep Disturbances in Adults." *Sleep Medicine* 12, no. 8 (2011): 773–79. https://doi.org /10.1016/J.SLEEP.2011.03.013.

Climent-Sanz, Carolina, Genís Morera-Amenós, Filip Bellon, Roland Pastells-Peiró, Joan Blanco-Blanco, Fran Valenzuela-Pascual, and Montserrat Gea-Sánchez. "Poor Sleep Quality Experience and Self-Management Strategies in Fibromyalgia: A Qualitative Meta-synthesis." *Journal of Clinical Medicine* 9, no. 12 (2020): 4000. https://doi.org/10.3390 /JCM9124000.

Climent-Sanz, Carolina, Montserrat Gea-Sánchez, Helena Fernández-Lago, José Tomás Mateos-García, Francesc Rubí-Carnacea, and Erica Briones-Vozmediano. "Sleeping Is a Nightmare: A Qualitative Study on the Experience and Management of Poor Sleep Quality in Women with Fibromyalgia." *Journal of Advanced Nursing* 77, no. 11 (2021): 4549–62. https://doi.org/10.1111/JAN.14977.

Dietch, Jessica R., and Ansgar J. Furst. "Perspective: Cognitive Behavioral Therapy for Insomnia Is a Promising Intervention for Mild Traumatic Brain Injury." *Frontiers in Neurology* 11 (October 2020): 1208. https://doi.org/10.3389/FNEUR.2020.530273/BIBTEX.

Gaeta, Anna Michela, Ivan D. Benítez, Carmen Jorge, Gerard Torres, Faride Dakterzada, Olga Minguez, Raquel Huerto, et al. "Prevalence of Obstructive Sleep Apnea in Alzheimer's

Bibliography

Disease Patients." *Journal of Neurology* 267, no. 4 (2019): 1012–22. https://doi.org/10.1007/S00415-019-09668-4.

Gehrman, Philip. *Sleep Problems in Veterans with PTSD-PTSD: National Center for PTSD*. U.S. Department of Veterans Affairs. 2020. https://www.ptsd.va.gov/professional/treat/cooccurring/sleep_problems_vets.asp.

Goldstein, Andrea N., Stephanie M. Greer, Jared M. Saletin, Allison G. Harvey, Jack B. Nitschke, and Matthew P. Walker. "Tired and Apprehensive: Anxiety Amplifies the Impact of Sleep Loss on Aversive Brain Anticipation." *The Journal of Neuroscience* 33, no. 26 (2013): 10607–15. https://doi.org/10.1523/JNEUROSCI.5578-12.2013.

Ho, Fiona Yan Yee, Christian S. Chan, and Kristen Nga Sze Tang. "Cognitive-Behavioral Therapy for Sleep Disturbances in Treating Posttraumatic Stress Disorder Symptoms: A Meta-Analysis of Randomized Controlled Trials." *Clinical Psychology Review* 43 (February 2016): 90–102. https://doi.org/10.1016/J.CPR.2015.09.005.

Kalmbach, David A., Andrea S. Cuamatzi-Castelan, Christine V. Tonnu, Kieulinh Michelle Tran, Jason R. Anderson, Thomas Roth, and Christopher L. Drake. "Hyperarousal and Sleep Reactivity in Insomnia: Current Insights." *Nature and Science of Sleep* 10 (2018): 193–201. https://doi.org/10.2147/NSS.S138823.

Mathias, J. L., M. L. Cant, and A. L. J. Burke. "Sleep Disturbances and Sleep Disorders in Adults Living with Chronic Pain: A Meta-Analysis." *Sleep Medicine* 52 (December 2018): 198–210. https://doi.org/10.1016/J.SLEEP.2018.05.023.

Nassan, Malik, and Aleksandar Videnovic. "Circadian Rhythms in Neurodegenerative Disorders." *Nature Reviews Neurology* 18, no. 1 (2021): 7–24. https://doi.org/10.1038/s41582-021-00577-7.

Nutt, David J., Sue Wilson, and Louise Paterson. "Sleep Disorders as Core Symptoms of Depression." *Dialogues in Clinical Neuroscience* 10, no. 3 (2008): 329–36. https://doi.org/10.31887/DCNS.2008.10.3/DNUTT.

Pickering, Marie Eva, Roland Chapurlat, Laurence Kocher, and Laure Peter-Derex. "Sleep Disturbances and Osteoarthritis." *Pain Practice* 16, no. 2 (2016): 237–44. https://doi.org/10.1111/PAPR.12271.

Riemann, Dieter, and Christoph Nissen. "Sleep and Psychotropic Drugs." In *Oxford Handbook of Sleep and Sleep Disorders*. Edited by Charles M. Morin, Colin A. Espie. Oxford University Press, Oxford: 2012, 190–222. https://doi.org/10.1093/OXFORDHB/9780195376203.013.0011.

Vaou, Okeanis E., Shih Hao Lin, Chantale Branson, and Sandford Auerbach. "Sleep and Dementia." *Current Sleep Medicine Reports* 4, no. 2 (2018): 134–42. https://doi.org/10.1007/S40675-018-0112-9.

Videnovic, Aleksandar, and Diego Golombek. "Circadian and Sleep Disorders in Parkinson's Disease." *Experimental Neurology* 243 (2013): 45–56. https://doi.org/10.1016/j.expneurol.2012.08.018.

Wu, J. Q., E. R. Appleman, R. D. Salazar, and J. C. Ong. "Cognitive Behavioral Therapy for Insomnia Comorbid with Psychiatric and Medical Conditions a Meta-Analysis." *JAMA Internal Medicine* 175, no. 9 (2015): https://doi.org/10.1001/jamainternmed .2015.3006.

Zeitzer, Jamie M., Leah Friedman, and Ruth O'Hara. "Insomnia in the Context of Traumatic Brain Injury." *Journal of Rehabilitation Research and Development* 46, no. 6 (2009): 827–36. https://doi.org/10.1682/JRRD.2008.08.0099.

16. Other Sleep Hurdles: When Insomnia Is Not the Only Sleep Disorder You Have

Allen, Richard P., Daniel L. Picchietti, Michael Auerbach, Yong Won Cho, James R. Connor, Christopher J. Earley, Diego Garcia-Borreguero, et al. "Evidence-Based and Consensus Clinical Practice Guidelines for the Iron Treatment of Restless Legs Syndrome/Willis-Ekbom Disease in Adults and Children: An IRLSSG Task Force Report." *Sleep Medicine* 41 (January 2018): 27–44. https://doi.org/10.1016/J.SLEEP.2017.11.1126.

American Academy of Sleep Medicine. "Narcolepsy-Sleep Education by American Academy of Sleep Medicine." 2020. https://sleepeducation.org/sleep-disorders/narcolepsy/.

———. "Advanced Sleep-Wake Phase-Sleep Education by AASM." 2020. https://sleepeducation .org/sleep-disorders/advanced-sleep-wake-phase/.

———. "Delayed Sleep-Wake Phase-Sleep Education by the AASM." 2020. https://sleepeducation .org/sleep-disorders/delayed-sleep-wake-phase/.

———. "Idiopathic Hypersomnia-Sleep Education by AASM." 2020. https://sleepeducation .org/sleep-disorders/idiopathic-hypersomnia/.

———. "Insufficient Sleep Syndrome-Sleep Education by the AASM." 2020. https://sleepeducation .org/sleep-disorders/insufficient-sleep-syndrome/.

———. "Obstructive Sleep Apnea." AASM Fact Sheets. 2008. www.aasm.org/resources /factsheets/sleepapnea.pdf.

———. "Parasomnias-Sleep Education by AASM." 2020. https://sleepeducation.org/sleep -disorders/.

———. "Periodic Limb Movements-Sleep Education by AASM." 2020. https://sleepeducation .org/sleep-disorders/periodic-limb-movements/.

———. "Restless Legs Syndrome." AASM Fact Sheets. 2006.

———. "Shift Work-Sleep Education by American Academy of Sleep Medicine." 2020. https://sleepeducation.org/sleep-disorders/shift-work/.

Caliandro, Rocco, Astrid A. Streng, Linda WM van Kerkhof, Gijsbertus TJ van der Horst, and Inês Chaves. "Social Jetlag and Related Risks for Human Health: A Timely Review." *Nutrients* 13, no. 12 (2021): 4543.

Davis, Joanne L., and David C. Wright. "Exposure, Relaxation, and Rescripting Treatment for Trauma-Related Nightmares." *Journal of Trauma and Dissociation* 7, no. 1 (2008): 5–18. https://doi.org/10.1300/J229V07N01_02.

McHill, Andrew W., and Evan D. Chinoy. "Utilizing the National Basketball Association's

COVID-19 Restart 'Bubble' to Uncover the Impact of Travel and Circadian Disruption on Athletic Performance." *Scientific Reports* 10, no. 1 (2020): 1–7. https://doi.org/10.1038/s41598-020-78901-2.

Merikanto, Ilona, Laura Kortesoja, Christian Benedict, Frances Chung, Jonathan Cedernaes, Colin A. Espie, Charles M. Morin et al. "Evening-Types Show Highest Increase of Sleep and Mental Health Problems during the COVID-19 Pandemic—Multinational Study on 19267 Adults." *Sleep* 45, no. 2 (2022): 1–13.

Nesbitt, Alexander D., and Derk Jan Dijk. "Out of Synch with Society: An Update on Delayed Sleep Phase Disorder." *Current Opinion in Pulmonary Medicine* 20, no. 6 (2014): 581–87. https://doi.org/10.1097/MCP.0000000000000095.

Sá, José F.R. de, and Sérgio A. Mota-Rolim. "Sleep Paralysis in Brazilian Folklore and Other Cultures: A Brief Review." *Frontiers in Psychology* 7 (September 2016): 1–8. https://doi.org/10.3389/fpsyg.2016.01294.

Ward, Elizabeth M., Dori Germolec, Manolis Kogevinas, David McCormick, Roel Vermeulen, Vladimir N. Anisimov, Kristan J. Aronson, et al. "Carcinogenicity of Night Shift Work." *Lancet Oncology* 20, no. 8 (2019): 1058–59. https://doi.org/10.1016/S1470-2045(19)30455-3.

Parting Words

Johnson, Benjamin S., Kristen M. Malecki, Paul E. Peppard, and Kirsten M. M. Beyer. "Exposure to Neighborhood Green Space and Sleep: Evidence from the Survey of the Health of Wisconsin." *Sleep Health* 4, no. 5 (2018): 413–19. https://doi.org/10.1016/J.SLEH.2018.08.001.

Koffel, Erin, Adam D. Bramoweth, and Christi S. Ulmer. "Increasing Access to and Utilization of Cognitive Behavioral Therapy for Insomnia (CBT-I): A Narrative Review." *Journal of General Internal Medicine* 33, no. 6 (2018): 955–962.

Population Reference Bureau. *A Demographic Profile of U.S. Workers Around the Clock*. September 18, 2008. https://www.prb.org/resources/a-demographic-profile-of-u-s-workers-around-the-clock/.

Reiss, Benjamin. *Wild Nights: How Taming Sleep Created Our Restless World*. New York: Basic Books, 2017.

Index

Index

Index